Helping Hooves
Training Miniature Horses as Guide Animals for the Blind

Janet Burleson

Helping Hooves
Training Miniature Horses as Guide Animals for the Blind

By Janet Burleson

Copyright © 2000 by Janet Burleson. All rights reserved.

Printed in the United States of America.

Published by: Rampant TechPress, Kittrell, North Carolina, USA

Editors: Robin Haden and Cindy Cairns

Production Editor: Janet Burleson

Production Manager: Linda Webb

Cover Design: Bryan Hoff

Illustrations: Mike Reed

Printing History:

May 2004 for First Edition

Special thanks to John Lavender, Robin Haden, Sharron Davidson, Dan Shaw and Don Burleson for their contributions to this publication.

ISBN: 0-9744486-0-5

Library of Congress Control Number: 2004098385

This book is dedicated to the memory of Amos Carson Lavender, my father.

Acknowledgements

Publishing a book like Helping Hooves requires the dedicated efforts of many people. Even though I am the author, my work ends when I deliver the content. After each chapter is delivered, experienced copy editors polish the grammar and syntax. The finished work is then reviewed as page proofs and turned over to the production manager, who manages the cover art, printing, distribution, and warehousing. In short, the author played a small role in the development of this book, and I need to thank and acknowledge everyone who helped bring this book to fruition:

John Lavender, for his expert operational management. And production management, including the coordination of the cover art, page proofing, printing, and distribution.

Don Burleson, the love of my life, for giving me the inspiration and assistance that I needed to complete this project.

Robin Haden, for her expert editing and content advice.

Dan Shaw, for his enthusiastic participation in the Guide Horse program.

Sharron and Karsen Motsinger, for their unselfish willingness to volunteer assistance.

With my sincere thanks,

Janet Burleson

Preface

When the opportunity arose to conduct a feasibility study into the use of miniature horses as guide animals for the blind, it was exciting to have the chance to apply my decades of horse handling experience to the task of training these tiny equines in the skills required to successfully allow blind people to go anywhere, with confidence, while using an equine guide.

Horses have served as an integral part of human existence for centuries by providing transportation, labor, recreation and companionship. Indeed, it was the horse that first lifted man from the cold rough earth and transported him forward into civilization. One could argue that the advance of mankind would have progressed much more slowly if not for the aid of the horse. As late as the 1800's, horses were an indispensable part of everyday life, delivering products and services and providing reliable travel companions for millions of people. While the twentieth century saw a decline in the use of horses, these noble beasts are once again entering the mainstream of the human lifestyle.

Is it farfetched to believe that horses can adapt to our modern lifestyle and continue to provide valuable services to mankind? This question, as well as my own burning desire to bring the horse back as a part of everyday life, led to an interesting experiment in training and using horses, albeit miniature ones, as "Guides for the Blind". This is the story of our work in reintroducing horses into human society, hopefully repaying the debt that mankind has owed to these most noble of creatures for some time.

Janet Burleson

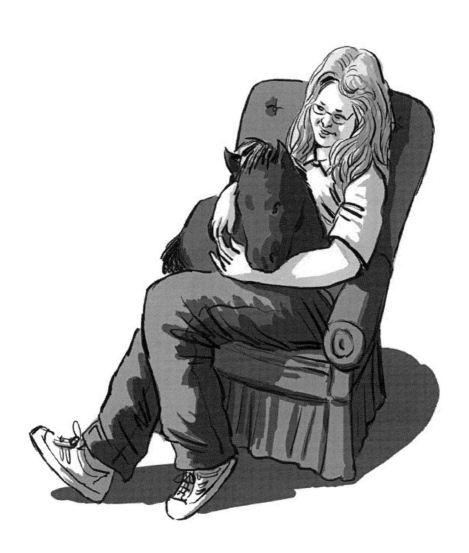

Horse Fever

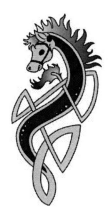

Mamaw, as my grandmother was affectionately known, helped to cultivate my affection for horses by telling stories of our ancestors and their bond with the horses that served them in day to day life. She used to sit me on her knee and tell me about her Grandpa, John Faulkenberry and how a noble war horse had saved his life at Gettysburg in the Civil War.

The Old War Horse

My great-great grandfather John T. Faulkenberry was a Confederate soldier. He served bravely in the Civil War with the famous Lancaster Invincibles. The Lancaster Invincibles, from

1

Lancaster County in South Carolina, were organized on the 8th of January 1861 and fought in many important Civil War battles including Manassas, Sharpsburg and Gettysburg.

John or "J.T." as he was commonly called, always said that he owed his life to his loyal steed "Rebel". He was said to have taken every opportunity to talk about his equine best friend. Obviously fond of his steed, J.T. even kept an old photo of Rebel with him at all times. Family legend asserts that Rebel lived to be over 30 years old. Great-Great-Grandpa is reputed to have mourned his death for decades afterwards, clutching his prized picture of Rebel as he laid on his deathbed, a grateful old man beholden to his loyal friend for giving him the chance to live a long, full life when so many of his Southern comrades-in-arms died tragically on the battlefield in the midst of their youth.

The following is John Faulkenberry's story as it has been handed down for over 139 years.

"I was only 19 years old when the war started and like all Sons of the South I was duty-bound to protect our homeland from Northern aggression. My daddy bought me three things, my pistol, a curved sword and the most prized possession of all, a spirited 3 year old gelding named Rebel."

Rebel was said to have been a stunning dappled gray horse with a fiery temper and fierce eyes that could look right through a person as if they weren't even there. Although small in stature, Rebel was a well muscled and sure-footed mount always steady in battle. John and Rebel became an inseparable team that fought together throughout the Civil War, including the harrowing battles of fighting at Antietam, Cold Harbor and Gettysburg.

The following are the family recollections about John's tales of his and Rebel's experience at Gettysburg:

"It was the second day of the battle, and it was unbearably hot and miserable. The noise from the cannon was deafening and all the while Rebel stood waiting peacefully until we received our orders. The Lancaster Invincibles were asked to flank the Yankees at Little Round Top and attempt to take the high ground. As we charged the bullets rained down on us like a hail storm and before I could even fire my pistol I felt a mini ball shove me back, nearly blowing me right out of my saddle. I knew I was hit bad, as blood was gushing from my shoulder."

At this point in the story, John was reported to have removed his shirt to show the massive red scars from the wound, much to the consternation and embarrassment of great-great grandmother Faulkenberry!

"I was on low ground, exposed like a sitting duck in the middle of an open field, dazed and losing blood fast. All I remember was whispering a fast prayer before slumping forward, to grab hold of Reb's neck so I wouldn't fall to the bloody ground. Next thing I remember it was dark and I was laying by a campfire safe and sound with no memory of getting there, I couldn't remember how Reb had saved my life.

I was told that once I was knocked out of commission Reb carefully turned around ignoring the hail of cannon and rifle shot exploding around him, he walked calmly from the field. They said it looked as if he was being very careful to keep me balanced in the saddle on his back as I lay there unconscious and limp like a wet dish rag. Even though he was wounded by shrapnel himself, Rebel carried me across the fields and through the woods all the way to the Regimental hospital before stopping to rest.

I reckon I wouldn't be alive today if it weren't for him."

The heartwarming story of a loyal horse like Rebel never fails to bring a lump to my throat even now. As a child, it definitely had a powerful effect that went a long way in making my affection for horses grow even stronger.

My first encounter with a real horse began with the family trips for milkshakes at Tony's Ice Cream Stand near Mamaw and Papaw's house. Tony's ice cream was homemade from a special secret recipe and was churned by an old sorrel gelding. This gentle soul walked around and around a beaten dirt track while harnessed to a shaft that turned the churn; technically speaking, I suppose that Tony's ice cream was "horse made" ice cream.

"Horse Made" Ice Cream

Every Sunday afternoon while the weather was warm, which is about 90 % of the time in southern North Carolina, we would go after church to visit Papaw and Mamaw in Lowell, a small mill town that was about a thirty minute drive from our home in the suburbs of Charlotte. The whole family would pile into our family size station wagon for the ritual trip to Tony's for the best milkshakes in the world.

We all loved Tony's milkshakes because after mixing up that delicious "horse made" ice cream with creamy cold milk and pouring it from the metal mixing cup into a wax drinking cup, Tony would plop a whole scoop of ice cream right on top of your shake!

He always gave you two straws because the shakes were so thick that one straw just wouldn't do the trick. You had to have a long handled plastic spoon too, so you could eat that scoop of ice cream in between the slurps.

Indeed, those shakes were a delicious and satisfying treat, but for me, it was seeing the horse that made those trips to Tony's so

4

special. When the gentle giant would take a break from his chore, we were allowed to visit with him. I would wait patiently in the parking area, under the shade trees, sipping on a strawberry milkshake watching Teddy steadily performing his task. All the while, I would be anxiously awaiting the opportunity to get close to that big, beautiful horse. He had large, dark expressive eyes that seemed to be looking right into your heart and hooves the size of dinner plates.

Papaw always spoke well of Teddy, *"Most people can't be trusted to work on their own the way that horse does."* He would say with an authoritative nod of his head in Teddy's direction. *"You can always depend on a good horse like Teddy to get the job done without messing around."*

Every so often, Tony would come out to stop Teddy and retrieve a batch of the freshly churned ice cream from his hard working equine partner's churn. This was my cue to run over to ask permission for a visit.

"I reckon it'll be ok for just a minute," Tony would say, *"But watch that you don't go sticking your fingers in his mouth,"* he would caution, *"Teddy's a real good horse, but he is a horse after all. He might mistake those stubby nubs for a carrot."*

When approached, the gentle gelding would always lower his head so I could stroke his well muscled neck. I would run my fingers through his flaxen mane which glittered like a pirate's gold treasure in the bright southern afternoon sunshine.

The best part was when Teddy would arc his neck around to touch my cheek with his soft muzzle as if to return the affection thereby giving me a chance to take in the sweet odor of his muzzle. Right then and there, I fell head over heels in love with horses and dreamed of climbing on Teddy's back for a gallop across the countryside.

Ever hungry to learn more about horses, I read the entire Black Stallion book series at an early age and lived, breathed and dreamed about horses. By age seven, horses were the focal point of my life. I collected horse models, horse books, horse pictures and the only thing missing in my life was a real, live horse. Believing that horses were only for rich people, I never had any expectation of actually owning a real horse but there was always the dream.

Oh Shenandoah!

Not long after I started grade school, Daddy was transferred to Virginia, which caused the family to relocate to the scenic Shenandoah Valley area. At first, moving and leaving our friends behind seemed like the end of the world, especially since the Virginia kids made fun of our Carolina southern drawl! But, the home our parents picked made all of the difference. It was a roomy split-level ranch in a new subdivision that was built on an old dairy farm. When the farmer retired, he had sold a large portion of the land for development, keeping his house and barn along with about fifty acres. By the time we moved there, he was running a horse boarding operation which involved renting out stalls in the old dairy barn and pasture space for horses belonging to the residents of the nearby subdivisions.

Living next door to a horse farm was the perfect situation for a horse crazy girl. I found the horses in the nearby pasture irresistible. I spent countless hours visiting with them and soon I could lead them over to the fence and climb on their backs. I would hold onto their manes for the ride as they moved through the pasture. With the help of these gentle horses, I learned to ride bareback in the most natural way.

After learning about my escapades riding bareback like an Indian, my parents were deathly afraid for my safety and instructed me to never enter the pasture again. Disappointed, I followed their wishes for as long as I could, but after a few weeks, the lure of the horses drew me back again. I was willing to risk suffering several rounds of punishment to be able to see the horses. To me, spending time with the horses was well worth the price. Fortunately, that wasn't necessary. My parents and I reached a compromise: I promised to keep up my good grades and maintain a clean room in exchange for formal riding lessons. Realizing how strongly I felt about being around horses, my parents decided that the best way to keep me safe would be to make sure I learned to ride and handle horses properly.

It was an exciting day when I went for my first formal riding lesson. The instructor assigned a chubby white hunter pony mare named "Snowball" to be my mount. She was aptly named since her coat was as white as fresh fallen snow. She had a big round hay belly that gave her the appearance of a big snowball with short legs and a fat neck with a tiny head. Unaware of the potential dangers associated with riding, I was fearless as the other four children and I mounted up and headed out around the riding ring to start our lesson.

The instructor stood in the middle of the ring amidst the white and red jumps and called out instructions to her pupils. *"Heels down!"* she shouted and we all shoved our heels as far down as physically possible. *"Heads up! Look where you are going,"* she reminded us because we were all now looking down to see if our heels were in the right position. After a few minutes of instruction at the walk, she felt we were ready to try the trot. One at a time, she told us to tell our ponies to trot a few steps so we could get the feel of our ponies' motion. This would give us the opportunity to start trying to rise up and down in the saddle in a coordinated motion known as "posting" to the trot.

Ever so confident, I nudged Snowball firmly in her well padded sides and she started off in a brisk trot. Unfortunately, I had not yet learned to guide a trotting horse as I was accustomed to riding on the backs of horses roaming freely in their pastures. As a result, Snowball had a chance to decide for herself which way to go, and she chose to trot into the center of the ring. *"Pull her back out to the rail!"* the instructor shouted. As instructed, I signaled Snowball into a left turn which just happened to point her head in the direction of a nearby jump. Being a well schooled and obedient hunter pony, Snowball naturally assumed that we were supposed to jump the little section of fence that lay straight ahead, so she lined up dead center with the rails and broke into canter toward the obstacle. *"She's gonna take that jump!"* the instructor warned, obviously alarmed that her beginner student would most likely fall and be injured.

Not knowing how to safely stop the accelerating pony, I just leaned forward and hung on for the ride as I had always done with the horses in the pasture. It was no different from hanging on and jumping the fallen log in the woods on the edge of the pasture. Snowball easily cleared the three foot high rails and cantered on across the ring.

"Easy girl, whoa, Snowball, whoa," I stopped the chubby white pony and rubbed her neck as the angry instructor strode over to us. *"What do you think you are doing?"* she demanded. *"You could have fallen off, Janet."*

"I'm sorry," I replied, too embarrassed to explain that it was Snowball's idea to take the jump. I thought it was better for the instructor to think I was an insolent child than to let her realize

8

that I knew how to stay on a horse while it cantered and jumped but didn't know how to guide it!

The horses roaming freely in the pasture had taught me how to enjoy their frolicking as a passenger. Now, a riding instructor would have to teach me how to harness the horses' natural energy and bend it to my will as a rider.

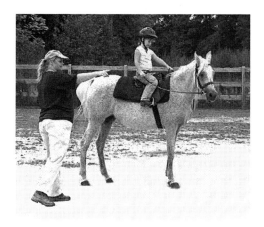

Surprise

That last day before Christmas vacation when Daddy came driving up to pick me up after school turned out to be a very special day indeed. As I was getting in the car, I noticed there was a saddle in the back seat!

Acting like nothing was amiss, Daddy said not a word about the well worn English saddle sitting on the red back seat of the white Ford Falcon. Dying to know what was up, I hesitated to ask, in case it was a secret. After all, it was the Christmas season, which for me was an extra special time as Christmas is my birthday, too. Finally, curiosity got the best of me, *"Daddy, why do you have a saddle in the car?"*

"Wait and see... just wait and see." He responded with a mischievous grin.

I didn't think I could wait until we got home, and then when he took a wrong turn, I was squirming in my seat with anxiety. We were headed in the direction of the horse barn, the "forbidden territory". Why would Daddy take me there? I assumed that he must have been dropping the saddle off for someone there.

Arriving at the barnyard, Daddy parked the car under a giant oak tree. He pulled the saddle out of the back seat as we climbed out of the car. We walked together into the old red dairy barn that had been converted to stable the horses. Stopping at the first stall on the left, Daddy sat the saddle on the top of the stall door and casually announced, *"Well, here she is, here's your pony."* He was pointing toward a young black pony mare peacefully munching hay. Absorbed in her meal of sweet smelling grass hay, the mare scarcely seemed to notice us standing outside her stall.

"No! Really?" In disbelief I hugged him quickly, *"Thank you!"* before rushing into the stall to visit with my new pony. Blackie and I were already acquainted as I had been riding her in the pasture for some time. She was only three years old and too green for her owner to handle. The owners had asked me to ride her in hopes that she would settle in, but her parents had decided to sell the pony rather than risk their daughter's safety. Knowing she was for sale, I had been wishing Blackie could be mine and now she was!

Daddy had finally accepted the inevitable and saved the money for the best combination Birthday-Christmas gift one could give to a horse crazy girl like me. Being thoroughly enamored with the protagonist in Marguerite Henry's popular book, *"Misty of Chincoteague",* I wanted to change Blackie's name to Misty. Mother suggested that since she joined our family during the Christmas

10

season, she should have an appropriately seasonal name. We settled on naming her Mistletoe with Misty as her nickname.

Misty and I became an inseparable pair that turned out to be quite a team. Together, we learned to canter on the correct lead and jump small fences in proper form. We even won a few ribbons in the horse shows. I learned far more from Misty than she learned from me as she taught me the basics of working as a horse's partner.

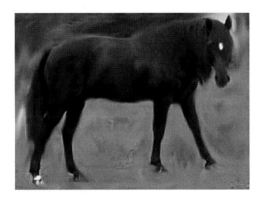

Runaway

The black pony mare pranced nervously and snorted as the growling truck closed the distance between us. *"Easy, Misty,"* I whispered with a sinking feeling in the pit in the bottom of my stomach. The narrow shoulder of the road provided a perilous path with a deep ditch to the right and speeding traffic on the left. There wasn't enough room to ride on the far side of the ditch to get away from the traffic as the steep bank went straight up to the barb wire fence line. When the monstrous dump truck came barreling down on us from behind, there was no choice but to stay steady and keep moving straight ahead.

With a roar, the rumbling truck was upon us and Misty bolted into a run like a thoroughbred that had just heard the starter's gun sounding the beginning of a horse race.

"Whoa, whoa, easy girl" whispering through the fear, I was just hanging on for the ride, terrified that Misty might unseat me. To the truck driver it probably looked as though the young gangly girl on the black pony was trying to out race the big truck. Indeed, the closer the truck came, the harder the pony ran as if it were a contest. Poor frightened Misty was running for her life. She had never before been exposed to such a huge noisy monster. Common horse sense told her to flee as quickly as she could to escape this predator. Normally, I would have turned her in a circle to slow her down and gain control over the situation. That just wasn't an option now as there wasn't room to turn safely. The only safe choice was to wait it out and focus on keeping her straight on the shoulder of the road while praying that she not stumble on the uneven ground.

After a few minutes that seemed like an eternity, the truck rumbled by leaving us behind. Realizing the threat had passed, Misty gradually slowed her pace to a leisurely walk. She settled right back down as if nothing had happened, but I was quite shaken. For me, this was one experience that would not soon be forgotten!

The next time a scary truck came along, I decided to dismount and hold Misty. My thinking was that it would be safer to make her stand and watch as the truck passed by. Upon hearing a big truck rumbling up the road, I swung quickly to the ground and stood in front of her. *"Easy girl, it will be OK."*.

Unfortunately, a frightened green-broke pony like Misty was not easy for a nine year old girl to hold. As the truck bore down closer, the pony began to dance and snort, whipping me about like a kite in the wind. Before I knew it, my feet were out of control and the ground rushed hard to meet the back of my head as the little mare knocked me down in her endeavor to again out race the noisy truck.

I wailed in pain as a hard hoof bruised my skinny shin bone. Determined not to lose Misty, I gripped the reins tightly with my fingers and I used my body weight as an anchor. This caused the pony to whip around to a stop, facing my prone body as the truck passed on its continuing journey down the road, oblivious to the havoc left in its wake.

Along with a few cuts scrapes and bruises, I gained a big dose of new found wisdom that day. As time passed, I would come to understand the importance of training a horse to "spook in place" sufficiently to control the natural flight instinct thus avoiding the danger of a runaway horse. After my injuries healed, Misty and I practiced dealing with frightening situations at home under controlled circumstances. This allowed her to learn to trust and follow my lead when threatened by something scary like a "pony eating" dump truck.

As I continued to learn more about horses and their behavior patterns, I decided that I wanted to spend all my days working with horses. An even greater opportunity to learn more horsemanship skills arose when our family relocated again to a sixty acre horse farm in the Shenandoah Valley of Virginia.

Lessons for a young filly

Shortly after acquiring Misty, my parents decided to buy a farm in the country where we could keep Misty and another horse or two. We moved from a subdivision to a sixty acre horse farm in the scenic Shenandoah Valley of Virginia. To my joy, the farm was located right next door to an American Saddlebred training stable. The impressive high-stepping Saddlebred show horses were a thrill to watch and soon the trainer was letting me climb on for a ride while he was cooling the fancy horses down after their workout. Riding these spirited horses was a dream come true for a young horse lover. These horses were so exciting to me! As the trainer came to realize that I had little fear of the horses, he let me ride increasingly more often until finally I was actually putting a Five Gaited stallion through his paces with ease.

One day while visiting the training stable, I noticed a young chestnut filly standing alone tied to the fence by the stable. The dainty filly was twisting her neck around pulling at the tie rope in an attempt to look back at the stable in search of her herd mates. She called out with the lonely heart wrenching whinny of a horse that wants to be reunited with its herd, then snorted and stamped her hooves.

Curious as to why this nervous horse was tied out by herself in the stable yard, I inquired, *"What are you doing with her?"*

"We're getting ready to break her," was the terse reply from the busy trainer as he brushed the glistening coat of a tall black mare standing tied in crosstie chains in the middle of the hallway of the stable. *"That's Cinnamon; she's an untrained two year old filly with a silly streak in her. Gonna let her stand tied out there today so she can learn that she can't always have her way."*

"She doesn't look that bad to me." I mumbled more to myself than to anyone else. I was feeling a bit put off by his cold response. Plus, like a lot of preteens, I believed I knew more than I actually did about everything. *"You don't know what you don't know,"* I always say looking back.

14

"Well, why don't you just go on and ride her then?" the trainer snapped, obviously peeved by my impetuous comment. Then he turned back to vigorously currying the horse he was preparing to ride.

Being just a kid, I took his suggestion literally and approached the frightened young mare. Offering my hand and voice to settle her nerves while blowing little puffs of breath towards her nostrils, I gave her a chance to know more about me and my intentions. Within a few moments, she was nuzzling my shoulder as I scratched her withers.

"You're a good girl, Cinnamon," I reassured her as she quieted down.

Using the fence as a mounting block, I slipped quietly across Cinnamon's back so that I was lying on my stomach putting just a little bit of my weight on her back. The rest of my weight was still supported on my left foot which was still firmly planted on the fence rail. Naturally curious, Cinnamon swung her head around and nuzzled my up-ended rear-end just as I decided it was time to slip off.

After a few repetitions of the less than graceful belly balance on her back, I slowly slipped my right leg over and sat upright on her back. She tossed her head a bit and I quickly slipped my leg back over and jumped down to stand beside her again. In this way, I was showing her that it was ok to let me sit on her back because I would be getting off again without doing her any harm. On about the third time that I sat on her back, the trainer came walking out of the stable and caught us in the act.

"What the devil are you doing child? Get off that horse!"

"She doesn't mind," I responded weakly, not understanding why he was so upset. Surely he would be pleased that I was helping with the filly's training?

15

"That horse ain't broke to ride." he declared as I quickly swung down and then back up again and quickly back down before the filly had a chance to spook or react.

"Well I'll be..." he mused, realizing that the horse was completely comfortable with a scrawny kid climbing on her back. *"Maybe you're on to something,"* he continued as he walked over to the dainty mare. While untying her lead rope from the fence rail, he asked, *"Mind if I lead her around a bit with you on there?"*

"Sure, go ahead. I can get off easy enough if she acts up." With a snug grip on her mane with my left hand, I was confident I could swing off easily, if necessary. There was no need to jump off as the little filly seemed comfortable carrying a rider. She walked quietly along as if she had been ridden bareback for her entire life.

"Well, that's amazing," the trainer commented later, with approval in his voice, after we had decided the filly had probably had enough work for her first day with a rider on her back.

Not realizing it at the time and quite by accident, I had discovered the basic principle of using the "advance and retreat" method of introducing a new concept or situation to a horse without causing it to feel alarmed. The very act of slipping on and off of the filly's back quickly gave Cinnamon a chance to adjust to the concept of carrying a human on her back without fear or force.

Cinnamon was the first of many horses that would learn this way as every horse that I had the pleasure of training to ride was introduced to a rider in this same manner. To this day, I always ride bareback first to allow the horse to adjust to carrying my weight in a comfortable natural manner before expecting it to carry saddle.

16

Another opportunity to pursue a new level in horse training came along with the birth of my younger brother, John.

Lessons learned from little brother

Always expecting to remain the youngest child of our family, I was both thrilled and surprised at age nine when my younger brother, John, was born. Since I was a handy babysitter, John was often left with me and I seized on this opportunity to share my horsemanship skills with him.

John was on horseback long before he was reliably potty-trained. When he was barely two years old, John was riding horses, using his diaper for padding with his little feet sticking straight out from the saddle. In no time at all, he had learned to trot and canter on horseback. At an age when most toddlers were still riding stick horses, John was charging along on a real steed, cantering through the hills and valleys of our Virginia horse farm.

As John grew older, he developed into an excellent rider who was accomplished well beyond his years and I couldn't resist enrolling six-year old John in a horse show class for riders who were 18 years old and under. He was quite a sight with his stirrups barely reaching the middle of his horse's side

The other riders' immediate reaction was *"Aww, how cute"*, but their tune soon changed when the shows began. John had hundreds of hours under saddle by this time, and he easily beat the older riders, posting in perfect timing and effortlessly guiding his fiery high stepping Arabian Hackney cross mare to win blue ribbon after blue ribbon!

Henceforth, little John was a force to be reckoned with, and his cuteness took second-place to his skills as a competitive equestrian.

John's story is an important part of the Guide Horse story because it was through working with him that I learned the importance of training horses to a suitable degree to work safely and reliably for someone other than myself. Training a horse to work for another handler or rider requires a higher level of attention to detail to ensure that the horse will perform as expected under all circumstances.

Back to Carolina

After spending just a few years on the farm in Virginia, Daddy was transferred once again, bringing the family back to North Carolina. Settling in the small town of Cary, we moved into a quiet older subdivision and were forced to board Misty in a public stable located a few miles away. It was tough being that far away from her, but I could make it to the stables in about an hour on foot or in half that time by bicycle so that I was still able to go riding every day.

In time, the inevitable "growth spurt" came calling and my legs grew too long to ride a pony, so Misty was replaced by a sixteen hand high Five Gaited Saddlebred show horse named "Please Believe Me" or "Please" for short. Misty went on to be another girl's special pony and my affections quickly transferred to Please.

The fiery bay gelding taught me there was a lot more to riding than slipping on the bare back of a pleasure horse in the pasture. Please was a real show horse and with consistent work he and I learned to perform together as a team. Unfortunately not long after we had reached the point where we could compete successfully in horse show competition, Please died unexpectedly from shock after getting cast in his stall during the night.

It was early in the morning on a school day in January as I was rushing to dress before walking to school when Mother entered my bedroom with concern showing in her expression.

"We have to go to the stable," she told me, *"There's something wrong with Please."*

"What is it?" I asked, alarmed at the possibilities, *"Is Please OK?"*

I knew that horses sometimes died suddenly from colic and I had once seen a foal die from pneumonia. Many scary thoughts were racing through my head.

"I'm not sure," Mother replied quietly. *"They called from the stable and asked that we come right away. That's all I know…"*

It was a tense quiet ride from our house to the stable that cold January morning. The fifteen minute drive seemed to take an eternity. Expecting the worst, I fought back the tears burning at my eyes. When we arrived at the stable, the vet was packing up to leave. He stopped his work long enough to intercept me as I rushed from the car headed at a run to Please's stall.

"I'm so sorry," he offered his condolences; *"there was nothing we could do to save him."*

"What happened?" I asked as the tears that I had been holding back now flowed freely. *"What's wrong with Please?"*

"We don't know for sure. He was in shock when they found him this morning at feeding time. It looks like he got down in his stall and couldn't get up. His legs were pinned under his feed box. We'll know more details later."

Please's death was an overwhelming loss, and it seemed like the end of the world for me. My special horse was dead, and I was never to find out exactly what happened. For the first time in years, I had no horse to groom, ride and love. Grieving and depressed, my interest in horses waned for the first time. Fortunately, my parents realized the lack of interest was only part of the grieving process, so they encouraged me to look for a new horse to fill the empty space in my heart.

For the Love of Arabian Horses

After the death of Please, my beloved Saddlebred show horse, I gained an interest in Arabian horses. The stable where we had boarded Please specialized in Arabians. Despite their small size, I greatly admired the Arabian horse's exotic beauty and fiery spirit. I was also impressed with the way they bonded so strongly with their human companions. Perhaps this bonding was a carryover from the days when the Arabian horses lived in desert tents with their Bedouin owners.

It was tough trying to replace Please as no other horse seemed to compare. After months of viewing and trying out prospective mounts, we visited a large herd of untrained Arabians belonging to Robert Peebles in Virginia. The prospect of starting from scratch with an untrained horse was discouraging because it meant that it would be a long time before we could venture into the show ring.

Mr. Peebles's horses were bigger than most of the horses we had considered so far and as a lanky 5' 8" tall teenager with long legs, that extra size was most appealing.

"Here's a nice three year old purebred mare by Fire Dance. Her name is Dancell," Mr. Peebles pointed to a tall bright red chestnut mare with a white blaze face and the teeniest bit of white on one rear leg down around the coronet band. Her mane and tail were short and scruffy and her brittle sun bleached hair made her look like she had been living out in the elements. She didn't have a small classic Arab head, but her eyes were big, dark and expressive. She was well built and looked like she had the heart to go on forever.

We all agreed that in spite of her rough edges, Dancell, whom we called "Danny", would be a suitable prospective mount. That left Mr. Peebles and Daddy to discuss the business portion and finally reach an agreement on price.

She was a fine athletic looking horse that offered great promise as a new mount, so I was happy with our selection; however, there was another horse in the pasture that was actively trying to attract my attention. The big bay mare kept following me around. She would touch her nose to my hands, touch my hair and generally just check me out. She had a large plain head and a thin neck, so we weren't really considering her at all.

"That one's just a half-Arab and she's only two years old," Mr Peebles informed us, *"You don't want to get a two year old cause you'll have to wait a year to ride her."*

"That's true, I wouldn't want to wait that long," I agreed, *"But I do like her personality. What is the other half of her breeding?"*

"She's out of a Hackney pony mare and by Fire Dance same as the chestnut mare so they are half sisters. Her name is Rudance."

"Really, a Hackney?" This information really sparked my interest since Hackneys are well known for their stylish high action trots and that was something I liked very much. *"Well, too bad she's not older! I would rather have her than the chestnut mare."*

As practicality outweighed fancy, we headed out of the pasture to make the arrangements to seal the deal on the chestnut mare. The bay mare, Rudance, followed me to the gate. She stood there looking longingly at me as we walked away. Then, she whinnied, and I stopped to look back at her. She was still standing at the gate nickering invitingly, so I walked back to rub her neck and let her touch my cheek in a proper goodbye.

"I wish we could take you home with us, girl," I whispered in her ear as she nuzzled my shoulder, *"Goodbye now."* I turned to go, fighting back tears as she continued to nicker.

"You really like that horse, don't you?" Mr. Peebles asked as I rejoined him and my parents.

"Yeah, she seems like a special horse. Maybe she reminds me a bit of Please," I answered with a twinge of sadness.

"Well," my father spoke up, *"we've worked out a deal here. We're taking both of the mares home with us. Mr. Peebles made me an offer I couldn't refuse!"*

"That's wonderful! Thank you!" What good fortune it was to be able to take the young bay mare home with us too!

In time and with steady consistent work, the young mares would both grow to be excellent mounts. But the bay mare, whom we nicknamed "Rudy", would prove to be a truly special horse that went the distance time and again. She became a multi-champion show horse and the mother of champions as well as a horse that even the smallest child could ride safely. To think we almost left her behind!

The years spent training Rudy and her half sister, Danny, helped me grow to be a well-disciplined horse trainer with the desire to make horses the core of my life's work. As a result, we leased a 28 stall horse stable about twenty miles from our home in Cary, NC and started a horse training and boarding business.

It soon became obvious the horse business wasn't all about blue ribbons and trophies. There were stalls to clean and hour after hour of riding lessons to teach. A typical day's work started at 7:30 am and ended at midnight. There was little time for anything but working with and caring for horses, but it didn't matter as long as I was working with horses.

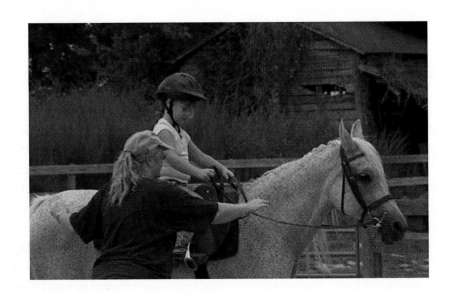

Karsen Motsinger takes a riding lesson on Vaalarie

Vaalor

Interested in starting an Arabian breeding farm, we contacted breeders across the country in search of suitable breeding stock. A respected veteran Arabian horse breeder named Darwin Allred from Missouri offered us a package deal for four breeding quality purebred Arabian horses. The package came at a bargain price and included one of the most stunning Arabian colts I had ever seen. "Vaalor" was breathtaking, with an exquisite head, a long, elegant neck like a giraffe and a tremendous *"look at me"* attitude. He was a son of "Excelsjor", a famous Polish Arabian stud who had been European Grand Champion Arabian Stallion as well as Swedish National Champion before being imported to the US. We could not believe that tremendous good fortune at having the opportunity to own such a beautiful Arabian stallion!

Over the years, Vaalor and I won numerous show championships. In fact, we won the North Carolina State Arabian Stallion Championship every time we entered. Vaalor always showed with an untamed spirit and the entire arena could hear his fiery snorting reverberate off the walls as he took the State Championship trophy. Vaalor died at home with me at the age of 26. Four of his children and several of his grandchildren still live with our herd of Arabian horses.

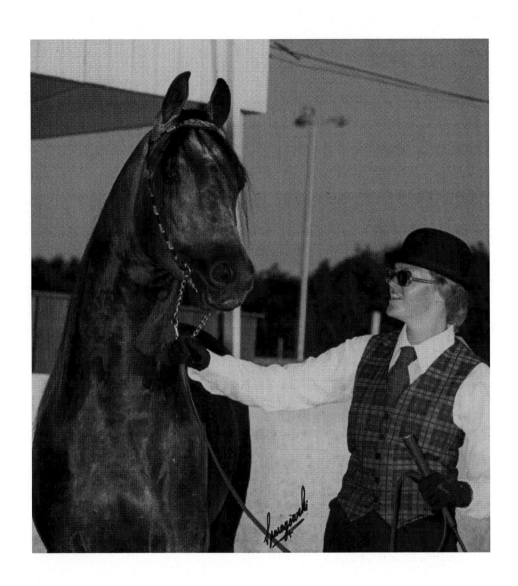

Vaalor

A New Lifestyle

After about twenty years of training show horses for the public, it was finally time to focus on other endeavors with horses. Specializing in training horses for others to ride in horse shows was rewarding work, but the downside was that it didn't leave much time to devote to my own mounts. Plus, having the ability to rehabilitate and retrain dangerously spoiled horses, I spent much of my time working with problem horses that could potentially hurt me! Lacking the invincibility of youth and no longer willing to face the risk of injury, I retired from professional horse training. After having had the pleasure of training a multitude of horses, from teaching initial manners to advanced performance techniques, I was anxious to focus more on the relationships between horses and humans rather than just training horses to perform basic repetitive tasks.

While content with my life's work, something important was missing. After spending years dedicated to the study and research of equine behavior and horse/human working relationships, it was painfully obvious that I had neglected to secure a balance in my personal life. It was time for a change.

Fortunately, one of my other interests opened the door to facilitate this change.

Something More

Horses had been my number one love for as long as I could remember. Little did I know; that was all about to change. It all started the day that I sent an e-mail question to the famous computer book author, Donald Burleson. Don's friendly reply came almost immediately which started a lively conversation as we emailed back and forth. Engaging in computer nerd dialogue, we discovered that we lived less than a mile apart. We quickly discovered how much we had in common and decided that we wanted to get better acquainted. Thoroughly intrigued by our conversations about computers, animals and art, it was exciting for both of us when we planned our meeting. It was a plus that Don's photograph in his books showed him to be quite handsome.

On the day we met, Don brought along his Cairn Terrier, "Chester", who despite being neutered, immediately began trying to seduce my little Yorkie-Poo, "Lizzie". It was love at first sight for all four of us. Easily embarrassed, Don was mortified by Chester's behavior, but we had a good laugh about it later.

Like me, Don was a lifelong animal lover with a driving interest in computers and animal training; we were a match made in heaven. We became engaged a few months later on Christmas Eve and were married the following June. The ceremony took place on the front lawn of our new farmhouse in Kittrell, NC on what had to be the hottest day of the summer.

Don has a degree in Experimental Psychology and studied for several years under the supervision of Dr Logan, one of the world's leading animal learning experts. His theoretical experience meshed perfectly with my practical experience. As a team, we were now ready to elevate my horse training efforts to a higher level. All that was missing was the right animal with which

28

to begin this work. Fortunately for us, a special animal would enter our lives through an unexpected path.

Enter the Ponies

After out-growing Misty, I never expected to own another pony. Then one day Don read a for-sale ad for a "miniature horse" in the newspaper. We were intrigued by the thought of adding a tiny horse to our growing herd.

"It would be fun to have a mini horse in the yard," Don mused. *"Let's go take a look but we don't want to rush into anything. We'll just look and then come home and let him think we aren't interested. Then maybe we can make an offer tomorrow and get a good deal."*

"Sure, let's just look," I agreed.

We drove an hour and a half to see the tiny bay pony named "Smokey", who was only about 30 inches tall. He was an adorably perfect little horse, so small and cute. In spite of our original plans, we took him home that very day, forgetting all about any discount.

Smokey was too small to safely leave with our full-sized Arabian horses. Besides, he was a stallion, so he would require separate housing. Since horses are generally happiest in a herd situation, we has concerns that Smokey might get lonely. A bored and lonely horse can be troublesome, and in true lonely horse fashion, Smokey soon began showing his skill as an escape artist. Early one 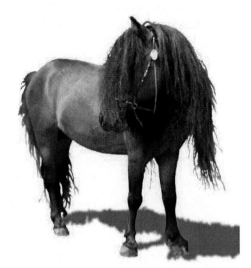 sunny Sunday morning, we went out to Smokey's barn to feed him, only to find the stall empty and the door wide open and swinging in the spring morning breeze. The latch wasn't broken, so how did he get out?

Having used the same clasps on stall doors and gates for large horses for 30 years without an escape, it seemed unlikely that Smokey had liberated himself! Alarmed at the thought of Smokey being stolen, Don immediately called the Franklin County Sheriff Department to report that a horse thief had visited us during the night.

While we were waiting for the Deputy Sheriff to arrive, one of our neighbors drove up in a buckboard wagon pulled by two Hackney ponies and told us *"I saw your little horse over in that field right after sunrise".* He pointed to the field across the road from our house. *"I thought it might be too early to come knocking on your door, so I planned to let you know on the trip back".*

We were relieved that our baby had not been stolen, but after several hours of roaming, Smokey could be anywhere in a ten mile radius! Right about that time, two State Troopers arrived and we were really embarrassed at having to explain that we had discovered that the pony wasn't stolen after all.

The officers were great sports about it and offered to help on the "pony sweep". I'll never forget the macho State Troopers walking though the surrounding pastures calling *"Here Smokey, Smokey"* in a deep commanding voice. Fortunately, we soon found the naughty Smokey munching grass alongside a neighbor's pond.

With hopes that lock-picking Smokey would never make another escape, we double locked all of his areas.

It took him awhile to learn how to open the double locks, but one day Smokey escaped again. This time he managed to get in with "Ibn Vaalor", a big gray Arabian stallion, who had a reputation for being an aggressive breeding stallion with no tolerance for other male horses. Fortunately, Ibn treated Smokey as if he were a foal rather than a challenger, a gesture that Smokey found particularly offensive. Smokey would charge at Ibn, asserting his presumed dominance as a stallion, squealing in a shrill high-pitched tone and biting at Ibn's chest and legs clearly intent on fighting until the end. Ibn, who could have killed Smokey with a single kick, was remarkably polite, even when Smokey's bites began to draw blood. Ibn would simply trot away, leaving Smokey to follow in hot pursuit. It was truly a comical situation. Once they tired each other out, we easily retrieved the exhausted Smokey.

It was clear that in order for Smokey to be content, he needed companions that were his own size, so off we went to a mini horse auction in search of pals for Smokey.

At the auction, we were overwhelmed with the multitude of types of miniature horses and ponies that were offered for sale. There were elegant modern Shetland ponies, dumpy ponies with fat bellies, a full spectrum of colors and a variety of refined miniature horses. One thing I had quickly learned about Don is that he likes something different, something unique. The search for a companion for Smokey would prove this beyond a shadow of a doubt.

SOLD! To the highest bidder

Late that night, Don came running up to me and said *"you've GOT to see this! A consigner has just brought-in one of the strangest horses that I have ever seen."* She was literally five feet long and only two feet tall, with super tiny ears and an uneven blaze that wobbled down her forehead. She looked like a Dachshund, except in horse form, and she waddled like a duck. *"Isn't she amazing?"*, Don said. *"She's really smart, too. Just look at her ears"*.

"Those are ears?", I replied, trying hard to stifle a laugh.

"Yeah, yeah, she looks funny, but just watch her ears move. She's listing carefully to me."

Sure enough, this wiener horse did seem smart and affectionate, but I could not see ANY use for her. She was too small for a child to ride and way too squat to pull a cart.

"I've just GOT to have her!", Don said. *"It's not every day you see such a unique horse"*. Well, I could not argue with that. Don and I agreed that we would bid up to $500 for this strange-looking creature.

"Do I hear 500,500,500…?" The auctioneer's chant sang out.

"Yee-ah!" The spotter yelled as Don's hand crept upward.

"I've got 500!" the auctioneer celebrated briefly *"How about 550? Can I get 550? 550,550,550..."*

"Please let it stop here." I whispered quietly as the auctioneer begged for more bids. Don had promised to stop at $500.00, but I knew how desperately he wanted to own "Blue Twinkle", the tiny horse walking in circles in the sale ring.

"550!" The opposing bid rang out from the other side of the stands.

"ALL right! I've got 550. Do I hear 600? What about 600?" The auctioneer questioned Don directly. He nodded his agreement to the bid as I groaned.

"I've got 600, do I hear 650?"

"Yeah!" Don's rival called out without hesitation.

The auctioneer turned his attention to Don once more, *"How about 700? I've got 650. How about 700?"*

Don's arm must surely have been bruised from my grip on it as he nodded to bid $700.00 for the ridiculous looking stubby legged mare with a foot-long tail that dragged on the ground.

"700! Let's hear 750, 750, 750..."

"750!"

"Awww-right! Now we need 800!"

Once more it was Don's turn. He hesitated. After all, $800.00 was a lot to spend for a deformed and spayed mare. But she was unique and he just had to have her… *"800"* he called out with a nod.

"Oh brother" I moaned.

"850, 850, how about 850?" Finally, Don's rival hesitated. Don's heart quickened maybe this would be it! Blue Twinkle would be his!

"850! I've got 850, do I hear 900?" The auctioneer turned to Don once more. *"How about 900?"*

"Honey, please stop." I begged.

Don shrugged it off, *"900"*.

"I've got $900.00!" The auctioneer rejoiced. "900, do I hear 950? 950,950,950…"

Silence.

"SOLD! Right here for $900.00 to bidder number… 98. Number 98 for $900.00".

The little dappled mare trotted out of the sale ring.

Flushed with pride, Don turned and asked, *"What do you think? Isn't she the coolest horse you've ever seen?"*

"I think you're nuts!" I answered honestly.

"Hey, I know what I like. Besides, what other horses do you want to bid for?" Don asked.

"We should head home. After spending $900.00 on that horse we can't really afford to buy any others." I answered rising to leave the sale arena.

The auctioneer's singsong chant continued in the background as another horse was offered for sale. *"I'll go settle the bill. Why don't you go find your cute new horse?"* I offered with a smile turning toward the sale office. Satisfied, Don nodded heading for the barn to retrieve his treasure unaware of the profound changes his purchase would cause in the days ahead.

Purchased on an impulse Twinkie would prove to be much more than a pet. She provided the inspiration for the guide horse training experiment.

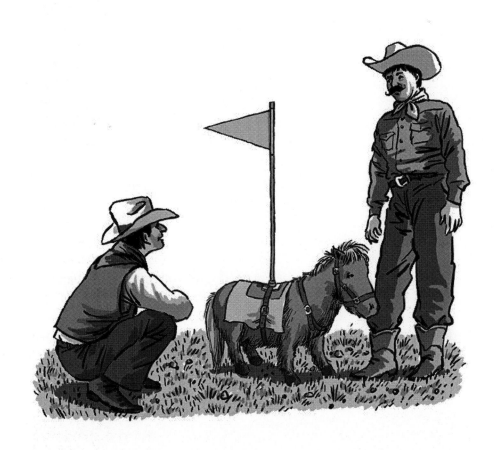

"It helps me find the little horses

in the tall grass."

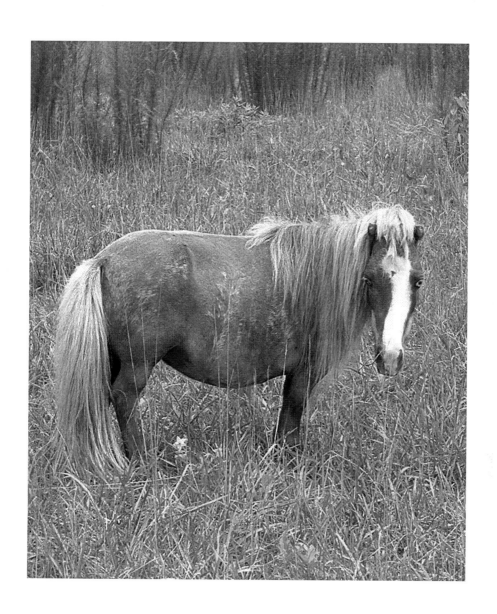

Wiener Horses

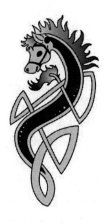

There was no doubt about it; Twinkie was a wiener horse, the Equine equivalent of a Dachshund, long and low.

Twinkie, the Wiener Horse

Standing only 25 inches high at the withers with a body the size of a much larger horse, Twinkie's head and neck were full size but her ears were microscopic, by comparison. They appeared almost as if they had been cropped like some dogs' ears are trimmed at birth.

Her legs were also true oddities. The femurs were significantly shorter than normal bones, proportionally, which gave the impression that she was missing portions of her legs. This unusual leg structure made her less than agile when moving.

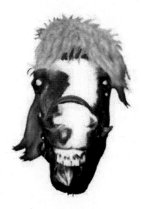

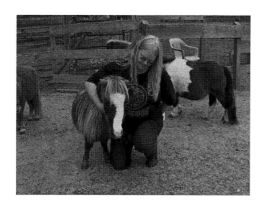

This was the cause of our present dilemma. We had seen other mini horses load easily into minivans as the little horses were apparently willing to jump right in. Twinkie, on the other hand, wasn't built for hopping into vehicles.

"Hey, need some help?" a passerby asked with a friendly smile. *"This little dwarf can be a real pain."* The muscular young man with tousled straw-like blond hair continued talking as he moved into position to help us lift the elongated pony into the back hatch opening of the green Dodge Caravan minivan.

"Did you call her a Dwarf?" Don questioned as Twinkie was boosted into her new means of transportation.

"Yeah, she was a normal looking foal at birth, but by the time she was three it was obvious she weren't quite right. The registry canceled her papers and said she's a dwarf horse."

"Really, was she your horse?" I asked.

"No, I brought her to this sale for my neighbor. She raised her from a baby and treated her like a spoiled pet. She had her spayed cause once she had a baby that was really deformed and only lived a few days."

"Oh my…" Don muttered sadly.

"Yep that was real hard on everyone, especially the little mare so Karen decided to have her spayed so she would never have to suffer like that again. She really loved that little horse but she can't afford to keep her any more."

"Well I just want her for a pet. " Don reassured him, *"She will have a good home with us."*

After saying our goodbyes and thanking the young man for helping us, we headed off toward home with our unique new herd member standing between the seats of the minivan with her head strategically placed between us. Twinkie made sure we had easy access to her head so we could provide her with plenty of affection during the four hour drive back to the farm.

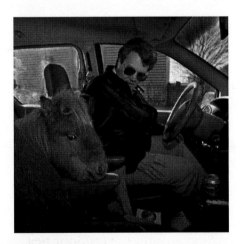

Ramping up

Don was so excited with the acquisition of Twinkie. He couldn't wait to show her off, so the next weekend, we took her to the Raleigh Flea Market at the NC State Fairgrounds. Since Twinkie couldn't get into the van by herself, Don enlisted the aid of our son, Andy, to make a ramp for her to use. Andy designed a portable ramp using four 1x6x48" boards covered with rubber gripping to provide traction so Twinkie's hooves wouldn't slip when she was walking on the ramp. The individual boards would wedge securely into the crevice of the side door frame of the minivan providing Twinkie with a steady surface for easy access to the van. When not in use, the boards were easy to store in the van as they could be stacked in a neat pile out of the way. Now we could take Twinkie anywhere!

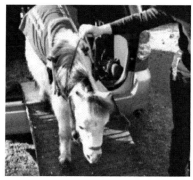

We removed the middle seat from the van and turned that part of the van into a rolling box stall with a tarp and shavings for Twinkie to use as a litter box while traveling. The kids, Andy and Jenny, sat in the backseat behind the horse much to Andy's consternation as Twinkie turned her rump his way just before dropping a big load of manure.

"Oh no!!! What the heck!" Andy screamed. Looking back, we saw him scrambling up the back of his seat trying desperately to get out of the way of the exploding manure bomb. Everyone laughed except Andy who did not think it was funny at all.

People are used to seeing dogs walking around the outdoor flea market with their owners, but a little horse like Twinkie stood out like a sore thumb. She attracted quite a bit of attention as she walked quietly beside Don as he perused the selection of antiques and collectibles on display. Patiently, Twinkie stayed close by his side as they moved from booth to booth weaving through the crowds of bargain hunters.

The dogs did not bother her although she upset quite a few canine companions. We heard a bit of barking and whining as they tugged on their leads trying to get a closer look at this unusual animal walking beside Don. The dogs were brave as long as Twinkie wasn't looking their way, but let her turn her head their way and they would yelp and run leaving her to wonder just what she did wrong.

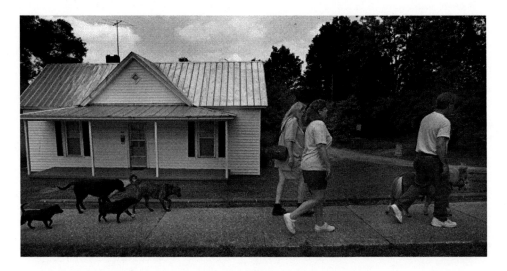

Twinkie surprised us all as she bonded with Don moving together as a team. *"Look how she handles these obstacles!"* Don exclaimed as she hesitated to navigate through a narrow passage, choosing instead to encourage Don to take a better path. *"She is guiding me like a seeing eye dog!"*

On the way home, we tossed ideas back and forth and all got excited at the prospect of experimenting with training Twinkie to be a service horse. Horses have a natural tendency to seek the safest path and to work as a team member, so a guide horse seemed to be a natural choice.

I also remembered, as a young girl, once watching a blind rider compete in horse shows. *"The woman gave the horse directions, and it took her around the obstacles and the other horses in the class,"* I told Don. *"It was serving as her guide horse while following her commands. That special delicately balanced relationship was something I have never forgotten."*

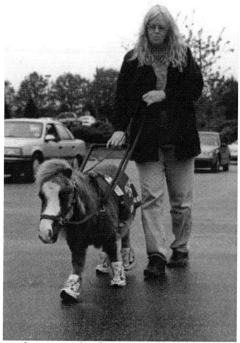

Impressed by the story, Don wondered aloud, *"Could a miniature horse like Twinkie be trained as a guide animal for the blind just like a dog? If there had been tiny horses available when people started using guide dogs, I bet they would have used horses without a moment of doubt!"* he said.

We already knew that horses have intelligence, strength, and stamina, excellent eyesight with a nearly 350-degree range of vision, and a superior long-term memory. Like I always say, *"Once they learn how to perform a task, they never forget."*

There were many complicated questions that had to be answered before we could seriously consider training a miniature horse to be a Guide Horse. One of the most crucial questions was whether or not a horse could learn to understand the safety issues involved when working in and around traffic well enough to effectively serve as a Guide Animal? While it would take many months of training and testing before we could feel comfortable that it was possible, a simple afternoon experience in New York City gave us the encouragement to invest the time and effort to test the theory.

The Horse Knows the Way

During an IT consulting business trip to New York City, Don and I decided to go horseback riding in Central Park. We were more than a little nervous at the prospect of riding unfamiliar horses through fierce city traffic that we weren't even comfortable engaging with a car. Hearing the concern in our voices, the young lady working at the rental stable was joking while trying to be reassuring.

"Relax," she said, *"These horses do this every day. They know the way to and from the park. You could even drop the reins, give them their heads and they will bring you back safely."*

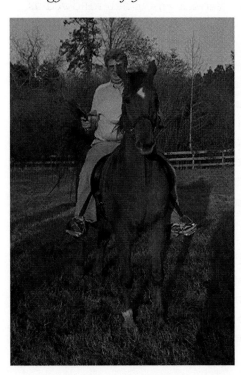

On the walk from the stable to the park, we noticed that the rental horses maintained a calm demeanor amid the chaotic Manhattan traffic. The animals also seemed to sense, on their own, when it was safe to cross the traffic path. They even appeared to understand the concept of looking both ways before crossing! Much to my consternation, I noticed on the return ride that Don was testing the premise that *"the horse knows the way"*.

"Honey! What are you doing? Pick up the reins… please." I asked, adding, *"You're making me nervous."*

"What? Can't I have any fun?" Don reluctantly gathered his reins and we made it back to the city stable safe and sound.

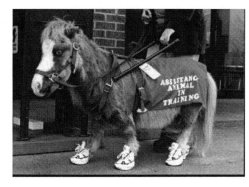

As a trainer of Arabian show horses for 30 years, I was certainly no stranger to the intricate nature of equine behavior. Even so, the urban street experience reinforced my thinking that we might be able to train a miniature horse to work as a service animal. This supposition held especially true for the affectionate and friendly 25 inch tall Twinkie, who often followed us around like a dog. This little horse was even right at home while riding in the back of the minivan like there was nothing to it.

Knowing that a great deal of work lay ahead in order for us to seriously attempt to train a service horse, we began to research the necessary behaviors. Beyond identifying these behaviors, we then had to devise a plan to instill them in Twinkie starting with basic obedience and response to simple commands.

Twinkie goes public

After we worked at home to teach Twinkie some basic commands and behaviors, we decided to take her to the Crabtree Valley Mall in Raleigh for a public training test. Don began working on a design for a guide harness for Twinkie. The building blocks that he used were a miniature horse driving harness and a handle made of PVC pipe.

Meanwhile, I sewed a blanket to designate her as an "Assistance Animal in Training" with little "Do not touch" signs to hang on the sides.

Concerned about the horse manure issue, we created a huge "Poo bag" from a 30-gallon trash bag that hung beneath Twinkie's tail. It was pretty ridiculous looking, but in theory it should have worked. Fortunately for us, Twinkie never tested the design as she just naturally chose to "hold it" while working.

The first time Don worked Twinkie in the Mall, we could hear passersby saying, *"Look a seeing eye horse."* as if they readily understood the concept. We were surprised at the warm reception by the public. It was as if service horses were a normal sight, and no one hesitated to accept the concept. Twinkie was so professional and well behaved while working that the Mall manager felt completely comfortable allowing us to test the Guide Horse concept there.

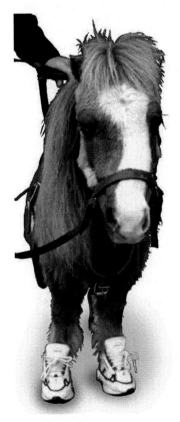

"You and Twinkie are welcome to train here anytime," the Mall manager assured us when we telephoned to ask permission.

This made all the difference in the world as the Mall was the perfect place to introduce Twinkie to a variety of stimuli and surfaces. The Mall offered crowds, noise, changing floor surfaces, ramps, steps, doorways, elevators, escalators and restrooms. These were new experiences for a horse fresh in from a life in the pasture.

Twinkie adapted easily to most of the mall conditions with the notable exception of the elevator. The first ride on the elevator was easy. She walked right in and settled in for the ride; however, when it started its descent, she felt the floor dropping for the first time and was a bit unnerved. It didn't help that the elevator had a back wall made of glass which allowed her see out into the mall giving her an open view of the mall background as we dropped down to the first floor! She behaved, in spite of her uneasiness, but the next time we wanted to enter the elevator, Twinkie didn't want to go in. She was convinced that we were making a big mistake by willingly loading us into this box that would drop down with us inside of it. She planted her little hooves firmly against the floor and flatly refused to budge in the direction of the elevator.

Since we realized and understood Twinkie's concerns, we used the *"advance and retreat"* horse training method to allow her to conquer her fear of the elevator. Twinkie and I moved away from the elevator and approached again. This time was different, however, because before reaching the point where she had balked before, I cued her to stop moving toward the elevator. This was followed immediately by a cue to head away from the elevator, in effect retreating from the "scary box". This time, we didn't go quite so far away before turning back to advance toward the elevator, succeeding in approaching a little closer to the elevator before retreating again. We continued to repeat this process and each time, on approach, Twinkie was a little more confident until she finally walked right inside the elevator.

We retreated a few more times, no longer going far away from the elevator. We just stepped in and out of it until she was no longer showing any concern about entering. We then practiced riding the elevator. We would exit and then immediately re-

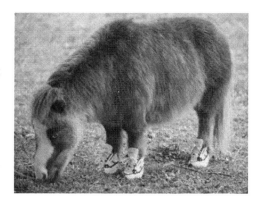

enter. We would ride to another floor and do it all over again. We repeated this five times until Twinkie was confident that elevators were safe. From that day forth, the elevator was an accepted means of transportation for Twinkie. She even succeeded in learning to find the button to call for the elevator when verbally cued to, *"Find the button."*

After we had put in a few trips to the mall, a local TV news crew asked permission to come along for one of our expeditions. Understandably nervous, we reluctantly agreed to be filmed for the evening news.

"Can you believe they are interested in our little experiment?" Don mused, *"Let's hope Twinkie makes us proud!"* Fortunately, Twinkie performed well as always.

It was from the filming of this newscast that we learned of Twinkie's need for additional traction on the slick floors in the mall. *"Her little hooves are slipping and sliding a bit in the back there."* The news anchorwoman stated while making slipping motions with her hands in the air.

The next day, Don invented horse sneakers! He created them by reworking children's sneakers. He cut off the heel portion and modified the shoes to fit Twinkie's hooves.

"This should do the trick. These shoes will provide all the traction she needs and they're cute too!" He announced.

At first Twinkie tried to lift her hooves out of the shoes, which resulted in her stepping in an exaggerated high fashion like a parade horse. She soon adjusted and appeared to appreciate the traction, if not the fashion statement.

The shoes were an instant hit with the public, eliciting comments like, *"look that dog is wearing sneakers… hey that's not a dog!"*

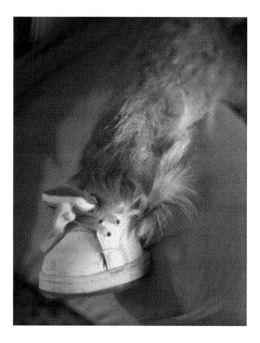

After completing the initial socialization and obedience training, it was time to start the serious guide horse training. Twinkie was an exceptionally dependable little horse, but would she be able learn the skills necessary to complete this experiment?

It was now time to take the training to the next level and begin serious investigation into the outrageous possibility that a tiny pony could work as a guide for a blind person. Next we explore the science behind the training if a guide horse.

OK, now signal
a left turn. . . .

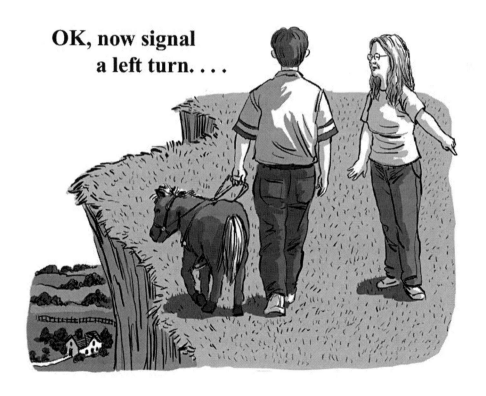

The Science Behind the Experiment

3

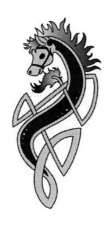

While it is a simple task to teach a miniature horse to follow specific commands and adopt desirable behaviors, guide work requires a more demanding level of training. The horse not only needs to be obedient and well mannered, but it has to consider all the factors within an ever changing environment and make split second decisions that can make the difference between safety and injury for the blind handler.

There are times when the Guide Horse must make the choice to ignore the commands issued by its handler and choose instead to adopt the practice of "intelligent disobedience" in instances where passively following a command would put the team of Guide animal and blind handler at risk. Anxious to continue the Guide horse training experiment with Twinkie, it was time to analyze the feasibility of adequately training a tiny equine to do such an important job.

Foundation Built on Research

The immense responsibility of training an unconventional animal to fill this critical job made it necessary to research the proven methods already in practice for training Guide dogs. This research included the careful review of every available book, tape and video on guide animal training and handling so that we could acquire as much pertinent information as possible. It was also necessary to invest considerable time interviewing Orientation and Mobility specialists, Guide Dog trainers and Guide dog users in an effort to gain in depth knowledge of the practical needs of a guide animal user.

At first, some Guide Dog professionals were uncooperative because they were skeptical about the wisdom of trying a different mobility assistance animal. Fortunately, there were those opened minded few who were willing to help explore the possibility of another option for blind people. Without their contributions, it would have been difficult to move forward.

Learning the dog training methods was just the beginning. The canine training methods had to be modified to suit the special nature of the safety conscious equine prey animal. One of the biggest differences lay in the animals' responses to correction methods. As pack oriented predators, dogs normally respond well and continue to learn while being physically corrected for inappropriate behavior. Horses, on the other hand, tend to learn more efficiently in a calm non-threatening environment. This type of environment is best facilitated with the use of positive reinforcement while asking the horse to learn complex tasks one step at a time. This made it necessary to develop a training program that would present the horse with non-threatening cues to keep it focused on the job at hand thus preventing undesirable behaviors from surfacing.

54

Learning how a Guide dog performs its job wasn't enough, though. It was also crucial to the learning process to collect detailed information about the mobility needs of the blind individuals. To adequately train a horse to perform the necessary guiding tasks, it was vital to understand how the blind person uses the animal as a mobility aid. Not the least of was to understand how the blind person interprets the information the guide animal supplies about the environment and the obstacles encountered. It is necessary to understand how the team makes decisions while navigating unfamiliar territory.

Armed with this newly acquired knowledge of conventional guide animals and mobility issues, it was time to make an informed decision about whether or not a horse was appropriate to use as a guide animal.

The next step was to investigate the physical characteristics of dogs and horses to fully assess whether or not a horse might be suited to do the guide work.

Through the eyes of a horse

When choosing an appropriate service animal, it is best to look for a species that is naturally well-suited to handle the necessary tasks. Having developed as a prey animal that depends on its senses for survival, horses have the visual ability to identify potential dangers which is key to keeping a blind person safe. In some ways, horse vision is even better suited for safety purposes than dog vision. After all, a horse, in its wild and natural state, had to be able to spot life-threatening situations at a great distance. This allowed sufficient time to make changes and enable the horse and its herd to stay safe.

The horse, being a prey animal, has a wide field of vision. They can see approximately 350° around because their eyes are positioned to the side of the head. A horse can track separate objects on either side of them simultaneously or it can focus forward using both eyes together for binocular vision. This increased range of vision makes horses better able to watch for potential obstacles and dangers, especially moving dangers such as automobiles.

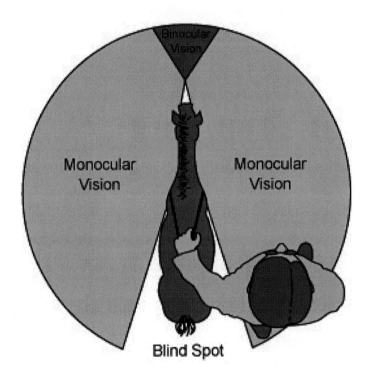

The phenomenon of binocular vision occurs when the visual fields of the two eyes overlap. Horses have a binocular range of about 65°, while dogs have a binocular field of 85°. In comparison, humans have a 120° range of stereo vision.

Dogs and cats can see about 150° around from their nose. As predators, their eyes are designed to be directed straight ahead so they can focus on their fleeing prey. Also predators, humans also have a frontal focus with limited side-vision.

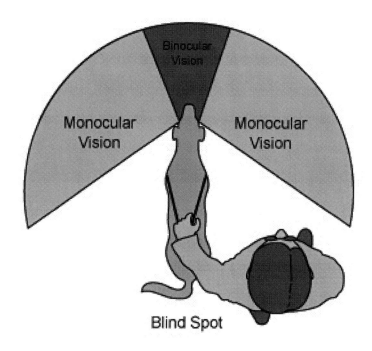

Unlike people and dogs, horses have the unique ability to track separate dangers with each eye. As horses evolved over millions of years, their brains developed the ability to simultaneously process images from each eye making horses capable of seeing potential dangers far better than people or dogs.

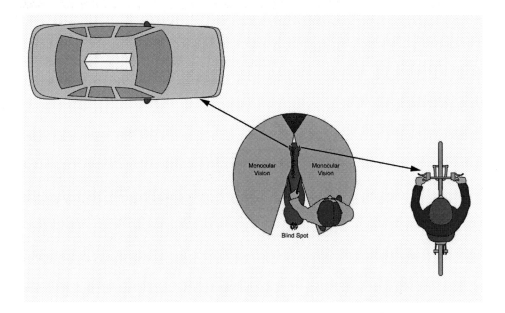

Through evolution as prey animals, horses developed extremely good night vision and can see clearly in almost total darkness. While a horse's vision during the day is better than its vision at night, horses see as well as owls and dogs at night. On moonless nights when we go out to feed the ponies, we can't see anything without a flashlight and they seem to know it. When in a playful mood they come up quietly behind us and then touch our backside, which always makes me jump! Then, satisfied with the effect of their prank, they offer a mane to hang onto so they can lead us to the feed bin so that we can serve their dinner.

In the popular movie *Seabiscuit*, there is a scene in which Seabiscuit is being trained at night in the dark in order to prepare in secret for the match with War Admiral. The half-blind jockey,

"Red" who is played by Toby McGuire, says *"I can't ride this track at night. I can't see a thing"*.

"Don't worry", replies Seabiscuit's trainer, *"He can"*, as he slaps the horse on the hindquarters sending him galloping off into the night.

It's true that horses see the world differently from humans. They lack a full range of color and have less visual acuity than humans, but their field of vision is much broader and is much better suited for night viewing. While very different in appearance from the human eye, the horse's eyes function quite similarly to human eyes in that they have good rotation ability, depth perception and eye-to-eye transfer.

While horses are not actually color blind, they do have a limited dichromatic color vision as illustrated in the comparison color wheels illustrated here.

Human Trichromatic Color Vision

Horse Dichromatic Color Vision

Comparing horse and human color vision.

In sum, horses are not color blind but have a limited range of color vision, specializing in the "nature" colors of brown and yellow tones.

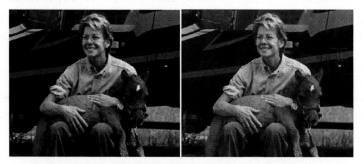

Human View Compared to a Horse's View

The photos above illustrate how a horse will view a common scene in comparison to a human's vision. Note that the colors are not as vibrant for the horse.

It is apparent that horses have the visual acuity to successfully perform as a Guide animal, but can a horse bond with a human to make a loyal working team?

Horse Loyalty

What follows is one of my favorite stories illustrating the undying loyalty a horse can have towards its rider. One weekend afternoon, one hundred or so North Carolina horsemen and women were enjoying the balmy spring weather while exploring the untamed woodlands when a bit of fun rapidly escalated to a life threatening situation. The story begins when the group encountered a man-made pond in a clearing where the riders stopped to let their horses wade into the pond to drink the cool water.

One young man happened to ride up to the opposite side of the pond from the others. Feeling the effects of a few beers, he carelessly didn't realize that he was approaching the pond from the dam side which generally doesn't have a sloping shore but instead just drops off into a deep water hole. At first the horse hesitated as if to ask the rider *"Are you sure this is a good idea?"*
The rider answered assertively while slapping the horse on the rump, *"Get on in there! It's just water, nothing to be afraid of."*

Having no reason to believe that the rider's judgment was in any way impaired, the trusting horse ultimately obeyed the command to enter the water just like the other horses were doing across the pond. Unfortunately, horses don't always understand the effect that alcohol consumption has on human beings!

From across the water, the young man's companions were startled to see him force his horse off the edge of the earthen dam only to plunge head first into the deep, murky water. Both horse and rider sank far under the surface where they were quickly separated amid violent splashing and desperate attempts to right themselves while striving to reach the surface.

The horse surfaced first and still focused on reaching the original intended destination, it began to swim calmly toward the opposite shore and the other horses. The rider, however, was still foundering under the water, obviously panicked and perhaps unable to swim. His hands repeatedly slapped at the surface, his head bobbed in and out of the water and then disappearing again as he sank deeper from the pull of his heavy wet clothing and boots.

At first, the other riders watched nonchalantly as they expected him to right himself and climb out of the water, so they were caught off guard as it became obvious he might drown if help didn't reach him quickly. They dismounted their horses to attempt a rescue just as the rider-less horse reached the shore and walked from the water, where she turned back to whinny and look for her lost rider.

Dripping wet and winded from exertion, the mare never hesitated as she immediately trotted back into the water and swam steadily toward her endangered partner. Upon reaching him, she slowly swam around him thereby giving him the chance to grab hold of her mane.

Once he had a secure hold, she slowly and carefully towed him across the pond and back to the shore where the stunned spectators helped him ashore.

If it hadn't been for those ten or so witnesses, no one would ever believe this to be a true account, but as the story spread like wildfire up the trail for the rest of the ride when that mare would pass by everyone would point her out as the horse that saved her rider from drowning before any of the humans could decide what to do!

Experiences like this one make it clear that horses can form unbreakable bonds with human partners to such a level that the horse freely chooses to take responsibility for the human's safety in much the same way that they look out for their equine herd mates and offspring.

Horse Guiding Instinct

In addition to their well suited physical abilities, horses are natural guide animals with an innate instinct to assist horses that are blind. Research yields an abundance of evidence that indicates that most horses have a natural instinct to guide.

Turtle Rock Rescue noted that one of their rescued Mustang horses named "Jess" assumed the responsibility of being a guide horse for "Pet", a blind horse. Jess takes the responsibility seriously even going so far as to ascertain that Pet has found the grain at feeding time before Jess will relax and eat her own meal.

Further research uncovered an article in the Equine Journal which noted:

> *"Horses are also natural guides. Cavalry horses were known to guide injured soldiers to safety. If a member of a wild band of horses goes blind, another horse often accepts responsibility to guide that horse. Many blind people ride horses on trails and in competitions, trusting the horse to lead them."*

In the book ***The Magic of Horses*** from Sunshine Press, there is the story of a blind cowboy named Gail Claussen and his use of "Shotgun", the Quarter horse stallion to guide him on his ranch in Colorado. From the book:

> *"Silk Shotgun is the seven-year-old, 1,300 pound muscled registered Quarter Horse stallion that Gail calls his "seeing-eye horse." Shotgun gets Gail out and about, and rather amazingly, Gail and Shotgun work the cattle together."*

Shotgun keeps this active cowboy mobile, and he gives Gail the chance to do what he loves, which is to work on the range. Yet it's not a one way street, for Shotgun, too, loves his work. If they need to round up the herd, Gail relies on Shotgun to tell him where the cows can be found. Once the herd is in Shotgun's sight, the horse turns his head in their direction; Gail feels it and knows where to ride. He and Shotgun then go after them.

He says that at times, he gets sick and tired of the inconvenience caused by his blindness, but when sadness threatens Gail, he drives it away with the help of his family, friends, and seeing-eye stallion. This cowboy tells it straight: "The outside of a horse is good for the inside of a man."

In *National Geographic Magazine,* there was a compelling story about a horse that saved a lost girl who was caught in a blinding snowstorm. She says that the horse "Arrow" saved her life by guiding her back home:

"My feet were numb and I thought I would freeze to death," she says. *"Finally I dropped the reins and let Arrow walk."*
Having only lived in the area for two days, Arrow was able to miraculously find his way back! Arrow and his rider were safe. Arrow now had a new home with his grateful rider.
"I don't know how Arrow did it, but he's a very intelligent horse who likes people," she said. *"He's my hero."*

Access Rights

Concern about possible access problems for a blind person working with a Guide Horse in public places mandated research into the laws governing access rights of individuals using service and therapy animals.

Surprisingly, it is obvious that the intent of the *Americans with Disabilities Act* (ADA) is to provide Americans with the right to use their choice of any "service animal" to assist with any disability. Non-traditional service animals are defined broadly, from leeches that help doctors re-attach severed limbs to the Capuchin monkeys that assist paralyzed people.

There is also the *Air Carriers Access Act* of 1986 (ACAA) which defines the regulations on commercial air carriers for those individuals who travel with their Service Animals. Learning that most major airlines have an Accessibility Department, I became involved with several of these organizations to help them understand the rights and responsibilities associated with the use of non-traditional service animals.

Historical use of Horses as Guides

Before society's divorce from horses, the guiding abilities of horses were very well-known by the general public. Perhaps if the Seeing Eye had miniature horses available when they first started training Seeing Eye dogs, they might have used horses as guide animals too.

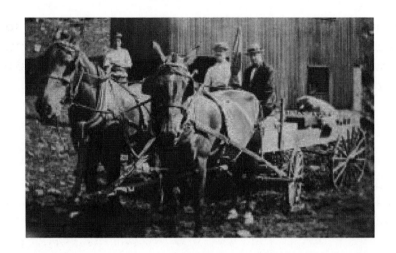

Horses could usually be trusted to find their way home unaided, and many a drunken farmer poured themselves into their buckboard wagons and slept while their horse took them home. As we know, dogs and horses alike make wonderful guide animals, and in some cases they have been known to work together.

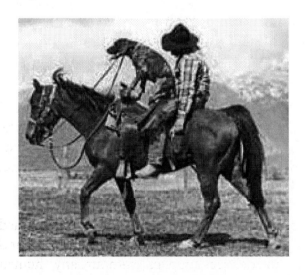

In Nineteenth century New York, cab drivers needed only to announce the name of the destination hotel and the Hack horse, having walked the route hundreds of time, would dutifully take the cab right to the correct doorstep.

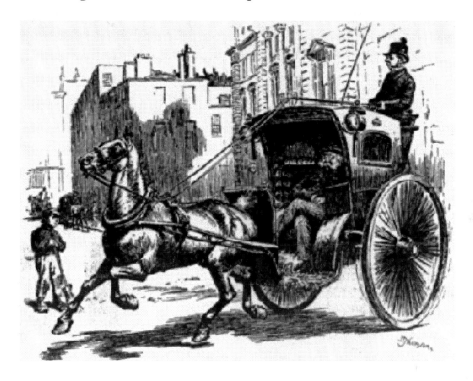

War horses were also well-known to be competent guides and many a wounded Cavalry soldier was carried safely from the battlefield on horseback. Such was the case in the experience of my great great grandfather during the Civil War when his horse, Rebel, carried him off the battlefield and back to safety.

During the Korean War there was a military horse named Sergeant Reckless who was famous for her calm under siege and her uncanny ability to deliver supplies without any human intervention. As told in the popular book *"Chicken Soup for the*

Horse Lover's Soul", Reckless would travel back and forth to the front lines during battle carrying supplies of ammunition to the troops. Sgt. Reckless was a loyal brave soldier dedicated to completing her duty no matter how difficult the conditions. She never faltered even when she was wounded twice in the line of duty.

Even with all this evidence of the suitability of horses for Guide work, many would still ask *"why use a horse"*? This is a legitimate question especially from those who were not familiar with the working capabilities of horses.

Why use a mini horse?

There are many compelling reasons to use miniature horses as guide animals. It has been shown that horses are natural guide animals and have been guiding humans for centuries. In nature, horses have been shown to possess a natural guide instinct. When another horse goes blind in a herd, a sighted horse accepts responsibility for the welfare of the blind horse and guides it with the herd. With humans, many blind people ride horses in equestrian competitions.

Some blind people ride alone on trails for many miles, completely relying on the horse to guide them safely to their destination. Through history, Cavalry horses have been known to guide their injured rider to safety. There are several characteristics of horses that make them suitable to guide the blind:

- **Long Lifespan** - Miniature Horse can sometimes live to be as much as 40 years old, with the average natural lifespan being 30-35 years. According to guide dog trainers, guide dogs have a useful life span of 8 to 12 years. These references to life span for both horses and dogs assume that the animal is given proper daily care and preventive and curative medical treatment, as necessary. In our own herd, we have two AMHA miniature horses that are over 35 years old and still enjoying life. The pair are still quite healthy and strong.

- **Cost Effective** - Training a guide dog can cost up to $60,000, according to the Guide Dog Users national advocacy group. According to Lighthouse International, there are more than 1.3 million legally blind people in the USA, yet there are only an estimated 7,000 guide animal users. Because of the longer working lifespan, a Guide Horse can be more cost-effective and ensure that more blind people receive a guide animal.

- **Better acceptance** - Many guide dog users report problems getting access to public places because their service dog is perceived as a pet. Most people do not associate a horse as a pet, and Guide Horse users report that they are immediately recognized as a working service animal.

- **Calm Nature** - Trained horses are extremely calm in chaotic situations. Cavalry horses have proven that horses can remain calm even in the extreme heat of battle. Police horses are an excellent example of well trained horses that deal with stressful situations. Guide Horses undergo the same systematic desensitization training that is given to riot-control horses.

- **Great Memory** - Horses possess phenomenal memories. A horse will naturally remember a dangerous situation decades after the occurrence.

- **Excellent Vision** - Because horses have eyes on the sides of their heads, they have an extremely wide range of vision of nearly 350 degrees. Horses are the only guide animals capable of independent eye movement and they can track separate potential dangers with each eye. Horses can see clearly in almost total darkness.

- **Focused Demeanor** - Trained horses are very focused on their work and are not easily distracted. Horses are not addicted to human attention and normally do not get excited when petted or groomed.

- **Safety Conscious** - Naturally safety oriented, horses are constantly on the lookout for danger. Horses have a natural propensity to guide their master along the safest most efficient route and demonstrate excellent judgment in obstacle avoidance training.

- **High Stamina** - Hearty and robust, a properly conditioned Guide Horse can easily travel many miles in a single outing.

- **Good Manners** - Guide Horses are very clean and can be housebroken. Horses do not get fleas and only shed twice per year. Trained horses will stand quietly when on duty.

Once we were comfortable with the relative benefits of using a horse as a Guide animal, it was time to start developing the step-by-step training process. The chapters ahead will share the details of the design and development of the Guide horse training program.

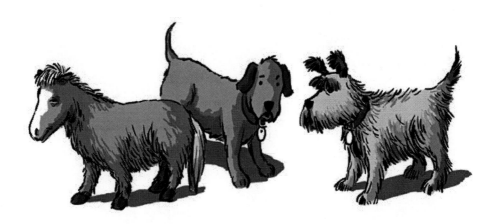

"Hey, Rover! Check out the tail on that puppy!"

Twinkie Learns
to be a Guide

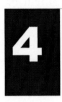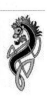

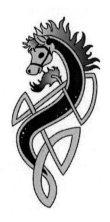

Encouraged by the prospect of developing Twinkie into a working Guide horse, we understood that she would have to master a variety of specialty behaviors before she could be effective as a prototype Guide horse.

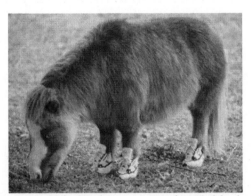

Twinkie had readily accepted the harness and quickly learned to lead forward of the handler while in harness. With practice, she learned the important skill of maintaining a straight line of travel while leading forward as long as the path was clear of obstacles. This was important because veering from a straight path would make it more difficult for the blind handler to remain oriented as to their location relative to their surroundings.

Once Twinkie was moving "Forward" on command and traveling in straight lines, it was time to focus on teaching her to respond to requests for changes in gait. The "Forward" command was her cue to move forward at an appropriate pace for the relevant conditions; however, it would sometimes be necessary to travel faster to cross a busy intersection or to cover a safe open expanse in a minimum amount of time. As a result, it was appropriate to introduce the "Faster" command as a cue to pick up the pace as long as it was safe for the team to move faster.

It was easy for Twinkie to learn to maintain the "Faster" gait until instructed to slow down with the "Easy" command, but more importantly, she had to learn to use her own judgment to slow down when necessary to keep the team safe. When crossing the street, it was important to move quickly until nearing the curb on the far side. Once safely across, she would slow down to alert the handler that they were approaching the curb. If the sidewalk had a ramp that did not require a step up, she could proceed at the slower pace without hesitation. If there was a step up or down, Twinkie would stop to alert the handler of the change in elevation before moving onto the sidewalk. In this way, the blind handler could tell they were nearing the side of the road as well as being alerted to the need to navigate over a change in elevation.

To enable the handler to control Twinkie with one hand, it was necessary to teach her to respond to directional commands instead of relying on guidance from a rein like a saddle horse. Twinkie quickly learned the proper response to the following commands: "Right"; "Left"; "Come About"; and "Back." Then she had to learn to find a suggested turn, "Take the next left" for example.

Getting Started

The first step in training a Guide horse involves introducing the horse to human companionship. The horses are often " as wild as deer" when they first come to the farm for training. Initially, socialization involves spending time with the horse and gently establishing a trusting relationship while maintaining a dominant position over the horse.

Once the horse is comfortable with being handled by humans, and the trainer's role as the wise "head mare" has been established, socialization becomes more complex as the horse learns basic manners and obedience. The horse should not fear its handler, but at the same time, it should have enough respect so that it does not view the handler as a play toy or a subordinate. As soon as the horse is no longer afraid of humans, it is natural for it to attempt to gain a higher position in the pecking order. This situation requires careful discipline to maintain the proper relationship between horse and handler.

To a horse, their human handler is either a leader or a subordinate. There is no such concept as peer in the hierarchical structure of equine society. Hence, it is necessary for the trainer to consistently control the horse's movements in early training to establish a position of gentle dominance over the animal. Once the horse recognizes the trainer as the benevolent leader eliminating the distraction of fear, true learning can begin.

For the potential Guide horse, basic socialization involves spending quality time with the horse. For a completely wild, untrained horse, touching its body all over is the first step, followed by lessons involving putting on the halter and leading the horse.

Advanced socialization involves working with the horse in public places and teaching it appropriate behavior in social settings filled with a variety of distractions and dangers.

When a little bay colt named Buckshot first came to us, he was terrified of people and so resistant to being near humans that when he was loaded via the side door into the minivan for the trip home, Buckshot panicked and leapt over the back seat and out through the open back hatch of the van. Fortunately, Don happened to be standing directly behind the van watching the events unfold, *"Whoa, little guy!"* Don said as he caught the flying foal in midair.

"Great save, Honey!" I called out relieved that we did not have to round up a wild pony running free across a fifty acre pasture.

"That was a lucky break," Don responded. *"Can you believe he did that?"*

"No, that was amazing! He just sailed right over that seat! Let's close the hatch this time." I slammed the hatch as Don placed the little guy back in the van via the side door behind the driver's seat.

After appropriate socialization, Buckshot settled in to become a friendly, people oriented mini horse.

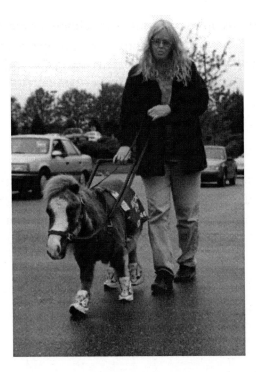

What does a Guide animal need to know?

Training any assistance animal requires an in-depth understanding of animal behavior as well as an understanding of the behaviors required for the animal to perform a service. Since basic equine behavior is generic to all horse breeds, any professional horse trainer can start the initial training of the assistance horse by teaching it to accept the harness, and start, stop and turn on command. Advanced training involves training the horse not to react to environmental distractions, to avoid obstacles and to recognize all potential dangers. The idea is to create a team with person and horse, working together, communicating and understanding one another in spite of the distractions they might encounter.

Guide horse Training involves the following areas:

- Basic Rein Training involves training the Guide horse to move forward at a speed appropriate for the prevailing conditions and respond to verbal commands while working on a loose rein.

- The Guide horse is also trained to negotiate everyday obstacles, including learning to enter escalators, elevators, climb stairs, and lie down on command.

- Voice Command Recognition: The guide horse is trained to respond to at least 23 voice commands, enabling the handler to direct and control the guide under any circumstance.

- Stationary Obstacle Avoidance: A guide horse must be able to alert the handler to obstacles in the path. Miniature horses readily avoid obstacles quite naturally, only needing to be taught that the handler is an appendage of themselves and how to communicate information about obstacles to the handler. In this way, the horse is taught to avoid low overheads and other stationary obstacles. The horse must be able to navigate sidewalks and streets, avoiding all obstacles, including any protrusions that may injure its handler.

- Distraction Avoidance: Guide horses must be able to ignore all distractions while guiding, and all Guide horses are thoroughly trained and tested to ensure that they will not "spook and run" while guiding.

- Moving Obstacle Avoidance: Once a Guide horse becomes proficient with Stationary Obstacle Avoidance, the training advances to the next level. This phase of training teaches the Guide horse to avoid moving obstacles that threaten to impede their path or present a danger to the handler. These obstacles include pedestrians, cyclists, motor vehicles, and any other moving object that may impede the progress of the handler. This is one of the most important areas of guide training as it deals with some of the most potentially dangerous obstacles that a Guide horse and handler team might encounter. Plus, the movement of the obstacles adds extra degrees of difficulty as the animal must not only be aware of the obstacle's presence, the animal must also anticipate changing conditions that could affect the safety of the handler.

Moving Obstacle avoidance is an area that is critical to the safety of the Guide team. Guide horses must demonstrate absolute proficiency in this area before going into service.

- Surface Elevation Change Recognition: This phase of training requires the Guide horse to recognize and signal the handler as they approach any change in surface elevation, including steps, stairs and curbs. This involves training the Guide horse to signal the handler and pause upon reaching any steps or curbs, thus signaling the handler that a step-up or step-down will be required. The Guide horse should always be positioned to walk ahead of the handler in a slightly shoulder in position with it's head and shoulders angled slightly towards the handler's path of travel. The handler learns to feel the horse's position through the harness handle to judge the severity of a change in elevation. By interpreting the horse's body position the handler can accurately time the point at which each step begins as well as anticipating when the elevation levels out again.

- Housebreaking: Despite common belief, horses do possess bladder control, and many horses develop the habit of eliminating only in a specific area. For excursions under six hours, the Guide horse can be relied upon to maintain bladder control. Just as dog owners are required to utilize pooper-scoopers, Guide horses on longer excursions can be fitted with a plastic lined pony panty that catches droppings and allows for easy quick disposal of waste products.

80

- Intelligent Disobedience: The Guide horse is trained to disregard any commands from their handler that would be unsafe for either the Guide horse or the handler. This is the phase of training where the horse is taught to rely on its best judgment to help keep the handler safe at all times.

After much study of working guide animals, we created the following list of desired behaviors for Twinkie:

- Responsiveness to requests for changes of direction (right, left, come about, back) as long as it is safe to do so.

- Identifying and signaling the location of the appropriate target when cued to find the next "right", "left", "inside" or "outside" opportunity..

- Avoiding obstacles including stationary, moving, and overhead obstacles like tree limbs .

- Alerting the handler of changes in elevation such as curbs, steps, rough spots in the sidewalk, and tree roots.

- Traveling up and down stairs at safe steady speed

- Avoiding or signaling the presence of potentially dangerous footing, such as ice, puddles, or mud

- "Finding" and indicating targets such as door handles, curbs, steps, elevators, escalators, tables, seats, and the minivan

- Allowing space for both horse and handler to pass through doorways and other narrow spaces

- Working close to the left edge of roads lacking sidewalks, and returning to the proper path of travel after navigating around obstacles

- Judging the safety of street crossings and refusing to go forward when cued if it is not safe to do cross.

- Crossing straight to the opposite curb as long as it is safe to do so.

- Avoiding vehicles pulling in or out of driveways, parking lots, side streets, etc.

- Avoiding "drop-offs", such as train platform edges or loading dock edges

- Following a designated person

- Waiting patiently while the handler is engaged in non-travel activity, such as working or dining

- Staying focused on task in the face of distractions, including food, other animals, and human attention

The more advanced areas of Guide horse training include:

- Walking up and down narrow, possibly slippery, indoor stairs

- Boarding and riding public transportation vehicles, such as busses, trains, subways, planes, and taxis

- Exercising "intelligent disobedience" in instances where the safety of the team is in jeopardy, such as in heavy traffic during street crossings

- Working on special elements in the environment, such as escalators and revolving doors

In the category of manners or tasks related to living in the human-built environment, Twinkie has achieved high marks on the following tasks:

- Responding correctly to basic obedience requests, such as "come", "heel" (walk on a loose lead at the left side of her handler), "stand", "stay"

- Accepting grooming and tactual contact on all parts of her body

- Respecting the space of humans and tolerating human patting and touching, even by strangers

- Indicating when a bathroom break is needed and waiting until an appropriate opportunity to eliminate is offered

- Eliminating on cue in appropriate locations

- Going without a relief break for extended periods of time, such as during long trips on public transportation lasting more than two or three hours.

- Playing with or mouthing only appropriate objects and "leaving" other objects alone

- Standing tied quietly for extended periods of time when necessary

- Eating, drinking, resting, and eliminating in unfamiliar places as appropriate at the handler's discretion.

- Tolerating being separated from her handler and left alone in a stall or on a tie

- Spending the night in hotels and other unfamiliar locations

Now that we had experimented with the basic guide training principles, we were ready to look at how to meld the training program to suit the needs of the visually impaired. This involved hundreds of hours of additional research and working closely with guide dog trainers, orientation and mobility specialists and blind volunteers.

Now with assistance from these valuable resources and a solid understanding of the task at-hand, we were ready to let Twinkie be tested guiding a blind person.

Karen Clark

5

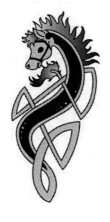

Now that it was clear that horses possessed the capacity to perform the job, we needed a blind person with Guide dog experience to help test Twinkie. Fortunately, our patience with the media attention paid off. We were soon approached by the perfect training partner.

Karen Clark

After being on the evening news a few times the guide horse story caught the attention of the producers of the TV show "Ripley's Believe It or Not". We soon received a call asking if we would let them film a segment on Twinkie for the show. By now we were getting used to being filmed. The first time you speak in front of the cameras you're a nervous wreck, the second time there's just a few flutters in your tummy and by the third time... well you come to realize that it's not such a big deal even if you do sputter and say things all wrong. So we readily agreed to participate in the Ripley's segment.

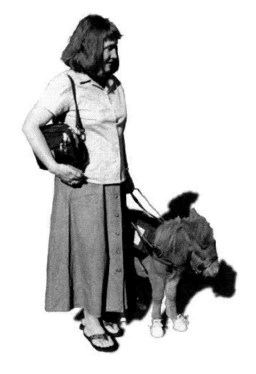

This was an especially important decision because the producer of Ripley's arranged for us to meet Karen Clark, a blind woman from Raleigh, NC who uses a guide dog.

Karen volunteered to walk with Twinkie to test the Guide horse concept. She was then generous enough to give us feedback from her perspective of the guidance the handler needed to receive from the animal. Karen's assistance gave us the boost we needed to be able to keep moving forward refining the training program.

Karen continued to work with us throughout the initial learning phase. She was happy with her guide dog and did not want a guide horse for herself but in Karen's words. *"It's important to provide many options for mobility so people can choose the one that works best for them."*

Karen walked successfully with Twinkie in a variety of settings. First she used Twinkie in the relative safety of the mall and later crossed busy streets in downtown Raleigh.

Twinkie Retires

Twinkie's training ended after we were satisfied that she had proven that it was feasible to train a horse to the level required to safely guide a blind person. We were now ready to move forth and train a horse that would be small enough to actually be used as a service animal. Twinkie was only a prototype and it was never our intention to use her as a working Guide horse because of the physical limitations associated with her special conformation. While her height was suitable the length of her body limited her ability to be accessible enough to adequately serve as anything more than a demo Guide horse. Her work completed, Twinkie returned to a life of leisure grazing and playing with her herd of buddies in a large open pasture on our farm.

It was now time to allow a blind person to participate in the next phase of the Guide horse training experiment. The challenge was to attempt training a horse for full time service. Twinkie could retire and we would start training a young horse that would potentially be placed into service as a Guide Horse.

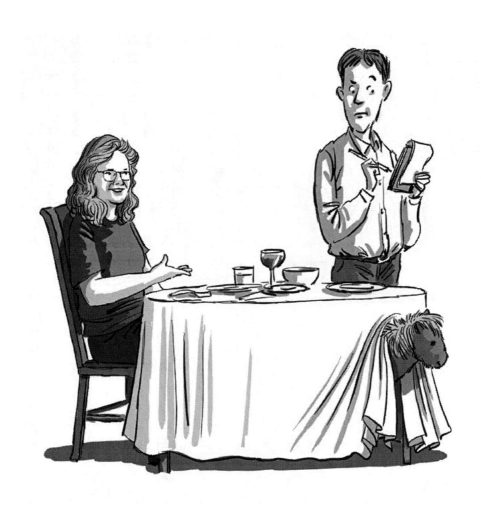

"And a large bowl of carrots please."

Cuddles

CHAPTER 6

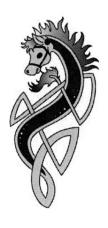

The next experimental subject was Cuddles, a dainty sorrel filly that showed the promise of staying tiny enough to be accessible to most public areas that the blind handler would want to visit. We started Cuddles in training as a young impressionable weanling before her habits were established. As such, it was easy for her to believe that all horses rode on escalators and traveled in minivans. Also starting young made it easy for her to accept the idea that there are some places where you do not go potty.

Lead Training

It was important for Cuddles to develop a firm habit of going forward ahead of her blind handler if she was to be an effective guide horse. We started ground driving her immediately instead of leading her so there would be no chance of her slipping into the habit of following her blind handler instead of leading. Two six-foot long lead lines were snapped to the side rings on Cuddle's halter for use as driving reins.

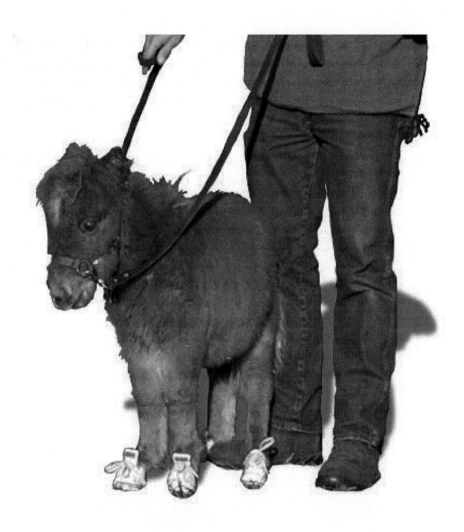

A six-foot long lead line was snapped to each side of the halter for use as reins to guide Cuddles.

Using the long lines facilitated walking behind Cuddles while driving her forward. It was a simple process to get her moving forward as she was still quite wild and inclined to run away from humans any way. She quickly learned to go forward in response to the verbal command.

We could then walk behind Cuddles and teach her to respond to the basic commands: "Forward, right, left, easy, faster and wait."

The long lines were useful in the first outings to teach her to turn and stop on cue.

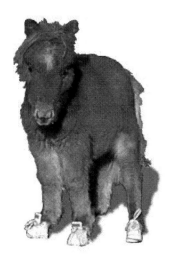

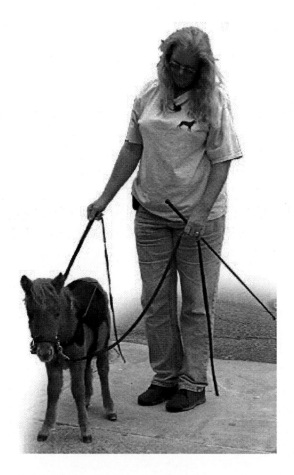

Part of Cuddles training was loading up into the minivan, and she would have to be very proficient at this task. Loading can be very difficult to teach a horse, especially when they must enter a tight enclosed area.

Starting out with a young guide horse prospect like Cuddles is basically the same as teaching a full size horse to load...

Load Up!

Brandi was a 16 hand blood red chestnut Thoroughbred gelding that had been converted to a Hunter after retiring from the track. A fun horse to ride with an owner named Sue who loved him dearly, Brandi came to our farm with various cuts scrapes and bruises he had received while being loaded onto the horse trailer when he left his old home. You see, poor Brandi had never been taught to load on a trailer and each time had been a little harder than the previous.

Now he had such a phobia of trailers that just leading him into the vicinity of the trailer parking lot would cause him to rear, strike out and pull back with all his strength. His owner was resigned to the fact that he was not going to be able to travel so when Sue was transferred to another state she felt her only choice was to leave Brandi behind. This was a heartbreaking decision because she could not afford to turn the job down just to stay with her horse but she did not want to try loading him as it seemed to be cruel to put Brandi through that battle again!

Brandi needed to learn to load up on command! Sue soon realized that leaving him behind wasn't the solution because Brandi would surely face the travel trauma again with his new owner. She then set out to learn how to erase her horse's fear and teach him to load up with ease and confidence.

The first step was to have Brandi feel safe while walking towards the trailer parking area. Since horses naturally use an advance and retreat method to investigate scary things, Sue started working on leading him toward the trailers then stopping and turning around to "retreat" just before reaching the point where he would normally freak out.

After a few trips back and forth she was able to gradually increase the "advance" stage so that the pair would get closer and closer to the frightening horse trailers without a reaction from Brandi. The first day's lesson had Brandi walking right up and touching the closed trailer without a struggle!

During subsequent lessons Brandi learned to walk up to the open trailer, then to step on the ramp, to ascend the ramp and back down, finally he was stepping into the trailer and backing out on cue gradually getting closer and closer to being fully loaded. By the time Brandi was loading completely he was comfortable and confident that he could walk in and back out properly without any problems or risks of injury. Sue now had a horse that would load like a pro simply because she was willing to give him the time to learn in small steps, advancing and retreating rather than trying to force him to jump in the trailer all at once.

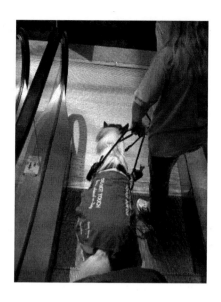

Escalator Training

We had never really considered teaching the horses to ride escalators until the day that nasty email arrived informing us that *"it's impossible to teach a horse to ride an escalator".* After that the challenge became irresistible so we set out to develop a method to teach the horses to ride on escalators safely and securely.

As it is a moving surface the escalator poses an unusual horse training dilemma. Ideally we wanted to let the horse step on one hoof at a time and back off gradually increasing the number of hooves on the escalator. But how do you do that with a moving surface? We soon learned that we while we wanted to give the horse every opportunity to advance and retreat sometimes we just had to enforce the "Forward" command sternly to get them on that first time.

Without fail, every new horse would have an accidental bowel movement the first time it was asked to ride the escalator no matter how reliably housebroken it had been. The escalator literally scared the poop out of them. On one such occasion when Andy and Jenny were helping with the training we had to clean up a high steaming pile that really embarrassed Andy. "Move along people nothing here to see." He told the onlookers, "Just some pony poop".

After that experience we designed the "pony panties" to catch the load in a training emergency.

Riding an escalator wasn't the only training topic that was discussed by the curious who did not understand a basic concept of horse training called de-spooking. During this training, a horse is taught to spook-in-place and freeze when they perceive danger. This is a fundamental concept in horse training and has been used for thousands of years, but has been lost in the 21st century as horses have faded from everyday life.

A spooky proposition

The Guide Horse Foundation uses the same techniques that have been employed for centuries in training Cavalry horses to remain calm, even in the heat of battle. The GHF also borrows techniques used by police departments in their training of riot control horses. The Guide Horses are systematically desensitized to chaotic and noisy situations and they are trained to ignore threats from other animals when in harness. Horses also look to their leader to know how to respond to a novel event.

In the horse industry this is known as the "lead mare syndrome". In a herd, all horses look to the lead mare to see how she reacts to a new event. If the lead mare does not exhibit fear, all of the horses will relax. This principle applies to Guide Horse training, and the Guide Horse will not exhibit fear if their trainer is not scared. A Guide Horse is required to "spook in-place" even when surrounded by chaos, and all Guide Horses must pass a test before being certified to guide the blind.

Crowd Desensitization

The State Fair presented the perfect opportunity to desensitize Cuddles to large crowds and loud noises with the diverse displays and bustling activity. She was a little trooper marching right along when noticing a section of rough ground around a large tree near the Lions Club booth I decided to test her ability to choose to use intelligent disobedience to protect me from taking a dangerous path. *"Forward, Cuddles!"* I commanded her to go forward towards a hole in the ground.

She complied moving out steady but when she reached the rough area she stopped using a shoulder block to prevent my stepping into the hole. *"Good girl! Thank you! Forward"* I asked her to move out again and this time she guided me around the hole, past the tree roots and on down the lane in the direction I asked her to go. "Miss," I felt a hand on my shoulder as one of the elderly gentlemen from the Lions Club booth reassured me, *"Miss, don't be angry with her she was just guiding you around a hole in the ground and some tree roots. She did an excellent job for you."*

Smiling I thanked him for his help and decided to leave it at that not wanting to ruin his moment of kindness by explaining that I was a trainer wearing black out glasses to test the Guide horse.

Because Guide horses would occasionally need to stay indoors for short periods of time, it was necessary to develop safety guidelines to prevent a curious pony from getting into trouble inside a house. While a toddler might learn about electricity by sticking their tongue into a light socket, I wanted to make sure that the horses did not have an opportunity to experiment with household hazards.

In the early stages of the program Cuddles was trained to lie down on command and to lie down under tables. This is a centuries-old technique used by horse trainers, most recently the famous Arabian gelding "Dervish" who appeared on the Tonight Show, lying down, covering herself with a blanket, and pulling-off a chain light.

Lying Down

In the early stages of the development of the training program we thought it would be important to teach the horses to lie down patiently for long periods of time. After Cuddles had mastered the "lie down" command we tested her by asking her to lie down and stay unattended for gradually longer periods of time while we were shopping. On one such occasion I left her lying on the floor of Belk's department store as I searched for an item near the far end of the aisle. Cuddles lay so quiet and still that a little old lady thought she was a realistic stuffed animal and poked her with her cane. *"My goodness! It's alive,"* she remarked pulling back startled as Cuddles raised her head and opened her eyes as if to say *"What? Can't you see I'm sleeping here?"*

100

Today, as horses are being used as guides for the blind, and to assist people with disabilities ranging from physically handicapped individuals to therapy animals, they need to learn proper indoor manners. Here we explore proven techniques for ensuring that horses that enter the indoor world of man are reliably housebroken.

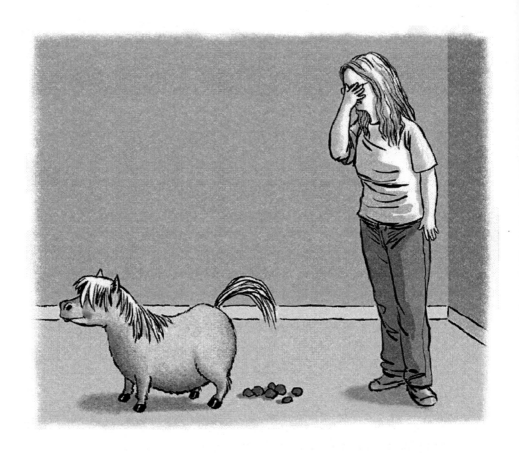

No..... I said sit!

Potty Time

7

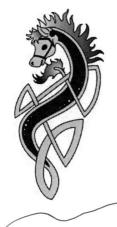

Unlike Twinkie, Cuddles did not wear a diaper during training, and she did not require any protection throughout her training. In the beginning, we encouraged her to go on pine shavings in a portable stall set up in the back yard close to our house. The shavings naturally encouraged her to relieve herself whenever she entered the stall. Taking advantage of this natural tendency, I would give her the verbal cue *"quiet time"* after releasing her in the stall signaling that she should relieve herself.

Once she relieved herself she was rewarded with a *"Good girl!"* followed immediately by a small food treat. After a few repetitions of this scenario she would go through the motions of relieving herself any time she was placed in the stall and told *"quiet time"*. During this period, I would reward her even if she did not need to go, thereby providing a solid positive reinforcement of the desired behavior. As she became proficient in her potty training, a scratching of the withers or simply stroking her neck replaced the food treat reward.

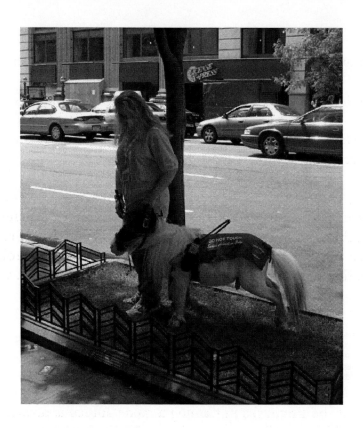

I've learned during years as a horse trainer that a behavior reinforcement can be verbal or artificial, as is the case with clicker training. Since I chose not to use the clicker training method, the *"good girl"* verbal reward was of the utmost importance as a verbal signal to the horse that it had found the appropriate response to the *"quiet time"* cue.

While using a clicker is an excellent way to signal impending positive behavior reinforcement to an animal, I found after trying both methods that a verbal signal of success is just as easily understood by a horse while not requiring any extra equipment that might encumber the teacher's hands.

The first steps with Cuddles housebreaking lessons were:

1 - Being placed in the "litter box" stall

2 – Using "quiet time" command to indicate that it was time to relieve herself

Next, it was time to move on to teach Cuddles not to relieve herself in inappropriate places. Nobody had ever attempted to housebreak a horse before, and frankly, I was not sure that a horse could be trained for long-term bladder control. But inquiring minds want to know, and I set out to see if it could be done.

Potty Training your horse

One of the first tasks in training a guide animal is housebreaking and initial socialization training. While I was familiar with housebreaking techniques for dogs, I was challenged to find a way to successful housetrain the mini horses, such that they could be taken anywhere without fear to an accident.

Here we will be discussing techniques that have worked for me in successfully training horses to be housebroken. There are two basic approaches to horse housebreaking, each suited to specific conditions:

Litter box method
Potty break method
The "bombs Away" method

To make the connection between being indoors and holding her bladder, it was necessary to take her inside the house and wait for her to need to relieve herself. During this time she had to be monitored constantly so I could catch her at the first sign of impending potty action, such a spreading her legs or raising her tail.

As soon as she showed a sign she wanted to go, we rushed out to the litter box stall where I released her while issuing the "quiet time" cue. Next, I waited while she relieved herself and then reinforced her with the "good girl!" verbal praise. It only took two repetitions of this procedure before she clearly understood that while inside it was necessary to go out to the litter box to relieve.

I had been successful teaching her to potty in the toilet, but was forced to abandon this method of training after discovering that health codes do not permit animals to use public restrooms. Evidently, the health departments feel that it is more sanitary for the animal to defecate upon the floor!

From that point on, I just had to watch for her to go to the door, and then immediately take her out to the litter box. After this became standard operating procedure I began to delay my response to her standing at the door so that she had to take a more aggressive action to alert me to her need to go out. I would pretend to ignore her until she began to paw at the door the same way a horse would bang on the stall door to ask for food or freedom. As soon as she would make noise with her hoof, I would then respond by taking her out to for a relief break. Using this technique, Cuddles quickly learned how to get my attention and how to make me jump up off the sofa!

Now that Cuddles knew how to let me know she needed relief, it was time to venture out into indoor public places. To do this, we needed a mobile "litter box" in order to maintain the continuity of the training experience. We made a rolling training stall with pine shavings in our minivan. When it was time to go on a training mission I would load her into the minivan, release her and give the "quiet time" cue. If she needed to go potty she would, otherwise she would just go through the motions in order to get her "good girl" reward.

After Cuddles relieved herself in the "litter box" there was a period of safe time before she would need to go again. During this safe time we could work on other aspects of her Guide Horse training while waiting for her to need to go potty again. During the safe time she could work indoors or in public places as long as we stayed close to the minivan so as to easily load her up if she needed to go.

It was imperative that she would make the connection between needing to go potty and needing to go get in the minivan "litter box". At home, Cuddles had learned to go to the door to signal her needs, and now she was trying to go to the door of a public building if she needed to take a break. At first I interpreted her tendency to go toward the door as a signal to take a break. After reinforcing this behavior a few times, I began to ignore her pulling toward the door, so as to force her to find a more obvious way to signal her needs.

This led her to fall-back on her hoof stomping action to let me know that she needed to potty. At the first sign that she was going to paw the floor, I immediately rewarded her with a *"Good girl"* and we high tailed it to the minivan for *"Quiet time"*.

Now that we had mastered the relief issue, it was easier to take Cuddles indoors and proceed with her advanced guide training.

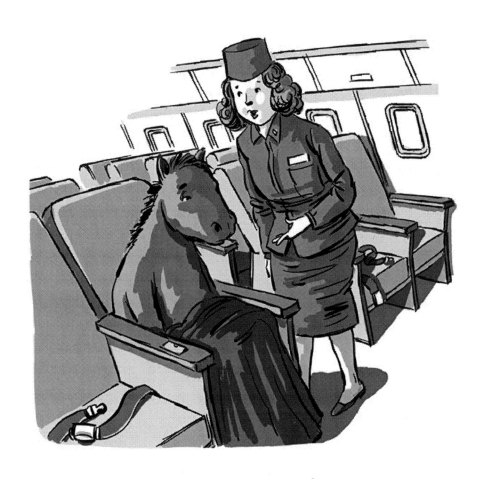

"Excuse me, why the long face?"

Pi Same long face!

Dan Shaw

 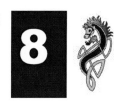
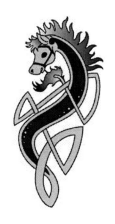

After several years of hard work and careful planning we were finally ready to start a full-time Guide Horse into service.

Dan Shaw & Cuddles were the first Guide Horse Team to be placed into full-time service. At home in Maine, Dan & Cuddles were united as a team in June 2001 and have been a successful working team ever since.

Back in the year 2000 Don and I were featured on **"Ripley's Believe It or Not"** on television and the blind people began calling. One especially insistent caller was Dan Shaw, a real pest who would not accept that we were an unproven and experimental program.

Dan recounts watching the Ripley's story. "I said to my wife, 'That is what I want. I'd be proud to walk down the street with a pony."

Dan Shaw is a 44 year-old ex-biker who sells fish bait and tackle in Ellsworth, Maine. I finally rewarded his persistence and we planned a rendezvous with Cuddles at the Raleigh-Durham International Airport to help him and Cuddles prepare for their new lives together.

It *"gives me tears"* to think about meeting Cuddles, Dan said. *"I just can't wait for the freedom of walking down the street with Cuddles,"* said Shaw, who lost his vision to an eye disease 27 years ago.

Dan is married with four children and 12 grandchildren. Of Cuddles, he said, *"She will be like family."*

Dan Shaw learned to expect a rough life from a young age. His parents divorced when he was 4, his father "ran off," and he moved with his mother from his home state Oregon to Lynn, Massachusetts. Then his mom remarried and went on to have four more sons. Dan felt like the odd man out as his stepfather was not particularly close with him.

Desperate for attention, Dan became a rebellious boy that had to be sent away to reform school for three years, *"and then I was passed around between different foster families."* But there was one happy summer that he spent at a camp for disadvantaged children; there he first discovered a new love, horses. *"I'd daydream about how I'd run off with one,"* recalls Dan, now 48 and a resident of Ellsworth, Maine.

Dan had learned at age 17 that he had an inherited eye condition, retinitis pigmentosa, which would eventually rob him of his vision. (His half brothers also had RP.) As if Dan did not have enough worries….

After marrying at age 19, his firstborn child was lost to crib death. Later he had two children, Danny and Jessica, but the marriage faltered. Angry that *"everything was not fair,"* Dan lived in denial. He wouldn't admit that he had trouble seeing because, he says, "people treated you different. They stopped coming around, they stopped being friends." Still a rebel in his 20s with tattoos covering his arms, he rode a motorcycle even as his sight slipped away. He bounced from job to job because he'd get fired when he messed up due to his vision problems, people thought he was drunk stumbling about. *"And still I was too proud to let anyone know"*.

In his early 40s when he had only 5% vision left, Dan realized he needed to prepare for a life of darkness. He attended the Carroll school for the blind near Boston, where he quickly began to read Braille so well that after graduation he began teaching Braille to sighted children *"so they could relate to what it's like to be a blind kid in school."*

But Dan's mobility problems in public continued, due to his proud refusal to use a white cane. In a restaurant he'd bump into a table and spill someone's drink; in a grocery store he'd stumble into little kids and incur the wrath of their irate parents. Eventually he was hesitant to go out at all. His second wife, was growing increasingly frustrated, tired of worrying about him while she was at work. *"He kept hurting himself to the point where I finally said, This is it—you need to do something now,"* she recalls. She had mentioned the idea of a guide dog before, but Dan resisted, he was an animal lover and couldn't deal with knowing of their short life expectancy. His wife persisted and he finally gave in.

As luck would have it one day in March 2000, they were sitting at the kitchen table filling out a guide-dog application with the TV on in the background. Dan caught the words, "guide horse for the blind." It was the Ripley's Believe It or Not program about the Guide Horse Twinkie.

"Hey," Dan said excitedly, *"that's what I want!"* He was especially excited to hear that the average lifespan of a miniature horse was 25 to 35 years, which meant he might be able to have just one for the rest of his life. He tracked down our phone number by calling Ripley's and became the first person to ask for a horse.

Dan volunteered, no he actually begged, to be the first guinea pig. We told him we were still testing the concept, but he pretty much talked us into going to the next step. We weren't ready to move forward placing Guide horses for full time service but Dan wasn't taking no for an answer. After much discussion and consideration of the risks involved we decided to let Dan work with us to test the Guide horse concept.

Dan's First Visit

After considerable pleading, pestering and general prodding, I finally let Dan come to North Carolina to see Cuddles. Dan was so excited that he could hardly contain himself when we brought Cuddles to the airport to meet his plane. Dan almost cried when he met her and a fast friendship was born.

We tested Dan's orientation skills with the Juno Walk, a procedure where the blind person walks with a guide harness handle attached to a human acting as the guide animal. Once we were convinced that Dan had the skills to navigate we decided to turn him and Cuddles lose in a crowded store. After a dew tentative steps, he immediately trusted Cuddles judgment and there was no stopping them. Dan and Cuddles tore around the store like two possessed maniacs, weaving between amazed customers and effortlessly navigating the crowded aisles.

For a tough biker dude, Dan was very emotional. As we loaded Cuddles into the car he burst into tears of joy, saying that this was the first time in over 20 years that he felt a sense of personal freedom. Suddenly all the work and sacrifice that we had invested was validated.

To this day I still get the greatest satisfaction from seeing how Dan regained his independence. Many of the blind people that we had interviewed during the initial research literally lived in darkness, a darkness of fear and self-consciousness. Many cloistered themselves in a cocoon and rarely ventured forth alone into the world.

For Dan, it was easy. All Dan had to do to meet people was to have a seat at a bench, and he was suddenly surrounded with new friends. We watched him patiently answer the same questions hundreds of time to curious onlookers and interested horse lovers.

On March 6, 2001 we flew Dan and Cuddles to Atlanta where they practiced riding escalators, elevators, moving sidewalks and people movers in Hartsfield International Airport. We also rode MARTA, Atlanta's rapid transit, to prepare for riding the subway in Boston, where Dan visits often.

"There has never been a horse on MARTA before," said transit system spokeswoman Kimberly Willis. But as long as Cuddles is serving as a "service animal" to Shaw, she is entitled by the Americans with Disabilities Act to ride MARTA, she said.

This was the first time that a horse had ever flown in the cabin of a commercial airliner and all of the media was there. We were surrounded by reported from ABC, NBC, CBS Fox and CNN, all waiting for Cuddles to misbehave. Of course, she was a perfect lady for the whole ride.

We had a wonderful time in Atlanta and we felt like celebrities, especially when onlookers could not see Cuddles on the moving sidewalks. Surrounded by cameras ad microphone booms, passerby's would exclaim, *"Who ARE those people? They must be really famous!"*

The only problem we had was Cuddles had stage fright. She had not gone potty for six hours and she was signaling me that she needed a break. We stopped at the outdoor relief area at Hartsfield airport, and six cameras focused on poor Cuddles. She froze and I insisted that the cameramen turn their backs to give the little lady some privacy! Once she was comfortable that no one was watching, Cuddles immediately cut loose, much to the amazement of all in attendance. She really was waiting for some privacy.

Road Trip

On the way home, we made stops in Washington, New York and Boston. Cuddles was the first horse to go to the top of the Empire State Building, Shaw said, and she will be part of a motorcade in Boston, where she will participate in a fund raiser for the Carroll Center and a graduation party for her and Shaw.

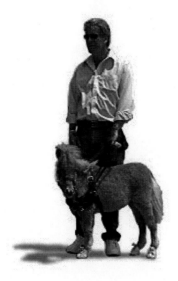

In Washington, Dan and Cuddles walked all over the Mall, visiting all of the monuments and impressing all who saw her. When we got to Manhattan we were relieved to find that busy New Yorkers saw nothing unusual about a mini horse guide in sneakers and we were welcomed everywhere. We rode the subway at rush hours, went to the top of the Empire State Building and took the ferry to the Statue of Liberty.

Cuddles was very impressed by the horse-drawn carriages in Central Park and we decided to let her have a ride. Dan gently lifted her into the carriage and Cuddles became the first horse to take a carriage ride in New York City.

Dean Irwin, the Emmy-award winning producer of the ABC 20/20 story about us invited us to the studio to meet Barbara Walters and Connie Chung. When Cuddles met Barbara Walters she sneezed, causing Walters to startle, making every laugh that the fearless political reporter was intimidated by a fuzzy pony. Later that night we visited Dean's penthouse apartment and Cuddles got to graze on the roof, gazing down on the lights of the city that never sleeps.

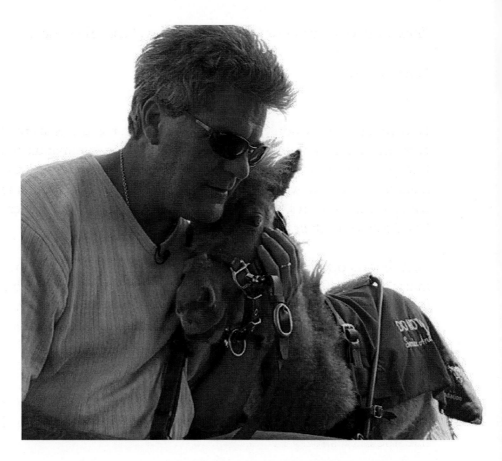

The Graduation ceremony in Boston was amazing. The sponsor donated a stretch limousine and we were accompanied to the graduation by a team of mounted police.

Hundreds of friends and well-wishers were there and the mayor of Boston was there to congratulate Dan and Cuddles on their pioneering achievement. The Dean of the Carroll Center for the Blind (Dan's Alma Mater) presented Dan's diploma to the thundering applause of the crowd.

"I can't believe the thrill that Cuddles has given me," Dan Shaw said.

"I feel normal."

Dan reports that Cuddles get better every year and has learned complex commands in addition to the 23 voice commands she learned in initial training. Cuddles can now respond to "find the mailbox", "take a walk" where she has memorized a walking route through Dan's neighborhood, and "find the car" where Cuddles locates their car in a crowded mall parking lot.

Dan reports one occasion where Cuddles saved him from serious injury. Dan & Cuddles were at an outdoor fair standing next to a large tent. *"There was a wicked fierce wind blowing that day."* Dan tells us. *"The tent was billowing and popping like it was alive but Cuddles never flinched. Then suddenly quick as a rabbit she moved me over away from the tent. At first I was angry thinking she was misbehaving... but then before I could reprimand her the whole tent came crashing down on the very spot where we had been standing just seconds before. My Cuddles saw it coming before anyone else did and saved us both!"* His eyes were moist as he rubbed the little mare's fuzzy neck in gratitude.

That wasn't the first time Cuddles sensed danger and forced Dan to safety. While Dan was in North Carolina training with Cuddles he was walking down the city street alone when a kid speeding on a bike on the sidewalk lost control of his bike when headed right for Dan and Cuddles. Dan didn't even know the threat was bearing down on him as Cuddles calmly led Dan off the sidewalk out of the path of the crashing bike.

Dan and Cuddles have also proven the practicality of Guide horse teams, traveling on long journeys alone and flying round-trip from Boston to Chicago to appear on the Oprah show. Unfortunately Dan's flight was delayed at takeoff and forced to sit on the tarmac waiting for an hour and a half. The extra added time made the trip too long for Cuddles to "hold it". Always reliable, Cuddles was distressed as the plane finally came in for the landing almost two hours late she whinnied loudly and dropped a few manure balls on the pad Dan had placed beneath her. The flight manifest described the event as *"The passenger in seat 22a had a bowel movement on the floor."*

Dan Shaw with Cuddles had demonstrated that a Guide Horse could mesh well with a rural lifestyle. Dan had a few acres for a barn and plenty of room for grazing. Dan told stories of his experience riding horses as a youngster at summer camp. The unanswered question still remained, could a Guide Horse fit into a suburban neighborhood lifestyle?

Just once, I'd like to choose
where we go today.

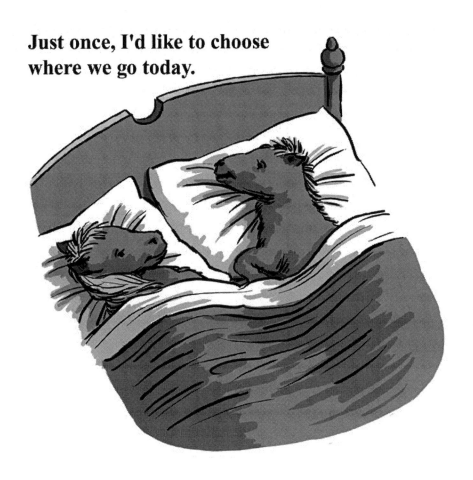

Tonto's Scout

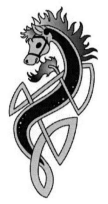

The question remains can a Guide horse fit into a suburban lifestyle?

Suburban Guide Horse

Shari is a homemaker in Pennsylvania where she cares for her husband Jim and their four boys, including a set of identical triplets. In December of 2003 she became the first person to experiment with having a Guide Horse in a Suburban neighborhood.

A lifelong horse lover, Shari was relentless in her pursuit of a horse guide. Shari passed her first interview along with an orientation and mobility skills assessment test when she traveled to the Guide Horse Foundation the summer of 2002 for preliminary work with Tonto's Scout, a talented two year-old blue-eyed Tobiano gelding , weighing in at less than 100 pounds.

A horse in the neighborhood

Growing up in PA Shari had always wanted a pony in spite of the fact that her family's urban home wasn't pony friendly. Shari talked of dreams about riding a pony for transportation around town since her vision prevented her from driving a car. Those childhood dreams fell by the wayside as Shari developed into an adult, married her husband Jim and became a mom to four wonderful boys, three of which were identical triplets.

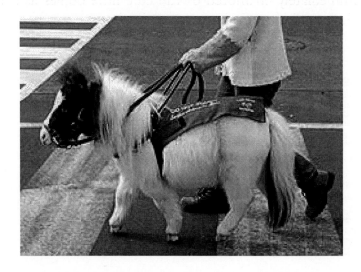

As the kids matured into teenagers Shari began to think of getting a guide animal. She hesitated to get a guide dog because of potential conflicts with the family pet German Shepherd Rio. Hearing about the Guide Horse program Shari thought she had found the answer to both her practical interest in a guide animal as well as her desire to work with and care for a pony. She filled out the online application and waited for the phone call that would signal the beginning of her participation in the Guide Horse program.

124

After several phone interviews, Shari was invited to spend some time at the training farm in North Carolina learning more about the Guide Horse program. This initial visit gave her a chance to learn first hand what it would be like to use and care for a Guide Horse.

Shari spent her first visit working with several different Guide Horses which gave us a chance to evaluate her ability to handle and care for a potential guide.

Shari was immediately enamored of the cute little ponies as she visited the farm for her preliminary evaluation.

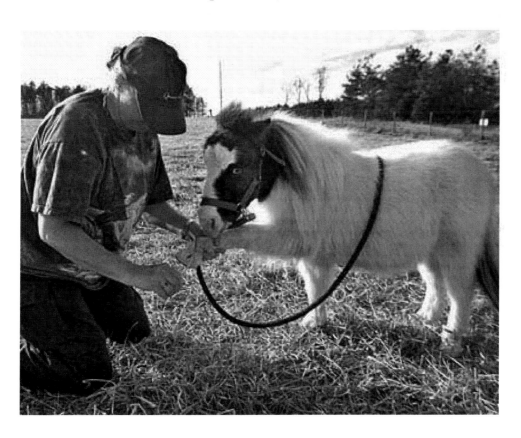

Just a few weeks before Shari was scheduled to come to the farm to train with Tonto's Scout, Don was traveling on a day long business trip to Manhattan. I drove him to the airport early that morning stopping at a grocery store in Wake Forest on the way home. It had been a long time since my last visit to the grocery store so the shopping list was long and the pile in the cart got higher and higher as I made my way thru the store.

"We have a bet going on your total." The cashier told me with a mischievous grin. *"Everyone's amazed at just how much you loaded in that cart! You must have a big family to feed."*

"No, not really," I responded smiling, *"just haven't had time to go shopping in a long time… the list just grew out of proportion."*

A Major Setback

It took two carts to carry the stuff out to the minivan but finally I was on the way home. It was a bright, clear North Carolina morning in February and all was right in the world as I set the cruise control to fifty-five miles per hour and joined the light flow of traffic northward on US Highway Number One. In twenty minutes I would be home on the farm spending the day working with the horses. Later I was planning to take Tonto's Scout with me on the return trip to pick up Don. A trip to the airport would be a good opportunity to work with him on the moving sidewalks and escalators. He could use some additional experience before Shari arrived to train with him.

In one breath everything changed as from the corner of my eye I caught sight of a car racing from a side road without even hesitating at the stop sign. There was no where to go as it hurtled into my pathway. For a split second it slipped from view and

126

relaxing with a sigh of relief I thought by some miracle it had missed ramming my vehicle.

Then *"BLAM!"* the unmistaken-able deafening sound of crunching and crashing metal filled the air as I felt the sudden impact agonizingly wrench my body. The van spun wildly as the airbags popped out slapping my face and throwing me backwards. I saw my left hand twist grotesquely as it absorbed the impact against the steering wheel. *"This is just not fair to my family"* raced through my mind as I believed death was near. It had been less than two months since we had lost our father to a heartbreaking battle with Alzheimer's, how could my Mother, husband and brothers deal with the loss of another family member so soon after Daddy's death?

Then the van slid to a stop in the road, *"It's over, I'm safe!"* I whispered mere seconds before a second impact sent the van air born off the road. At this point my vision had locked down to a tight field as I could not see beyond the airbag in front of me. Panicking and no longer certain where I was along the highway I feared the van might land in the nearby Tar River. Finally it came to a stop again as it landed in the trees on the side of the road. Dazed and frightened I tried to move my crushed left hand off the steering wheel but it wouldn't respond so I used my right hand to peel the useless fingers loose.

Terrified that the van would move again I frantically surveyed the trashed interior noticing what appeared to be smoke leaking in from the front floorboard amid all the rubble.

Releasing what was left of the seat belt I struggled to open the door but with the vehicle wedged between the trees it wouldn't budge more than half an inch. Frantic to escape before another impact I was trying to crawl to another door when I heard voices from outside the minivan.

"Are you OK in there? Sit still, wait for the paramedics." There were two men standing outside the driver's door.

"Please let me out!" I begged desperate to get away from the vehicle. I started pushing on the door again.

"Hold on, let's see if we can get the door open for you."

Finally they were able to bend the trees back and pull the door open wide enough for me to squeeze out so I could crawl away from the vehicle. Reaching the shoulder of the road I collapsed to wait for the ambulance.

The injuries from the wreck put the Guide Horse program on hold for six months delaying Shari's training until December instead of springtime as originally planned. Taking the horse home during the winter added to the difficulties of having a suburban Guide horse. The weather was nasty and Tonto didn't get as much work or exercise as he needed.

In spite of the challenges Shari put forth a concerted effort to bond with her horse in an honest attempt to learn to use him successfully in the suburban setting. She did an excellent job with Tonto but in the end outside forces interfered.

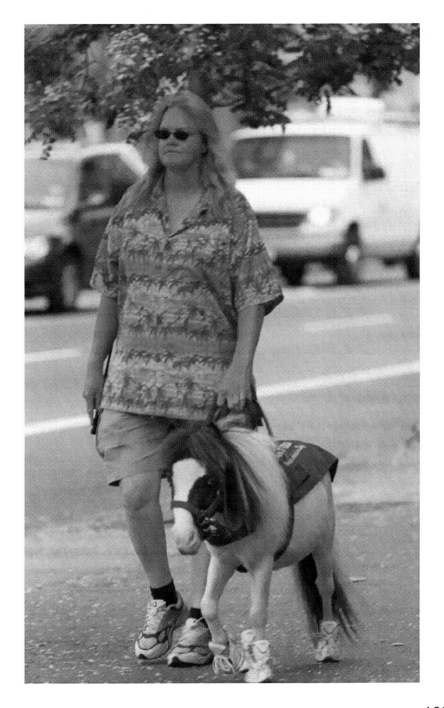

130

The Crusade

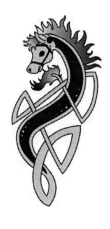

In early 2004 the training program was progressing well. We had placed three working Guide Horse teams, and they were all reporting that their guides were performing satisfactorily. We were encouraged that the program was showing success.

However, the peace was short lived. In March of 2004 there was a rash of misinformation on the Guide Horse training program published on a discussion forum on the Internet. It appeared that there was a group of people who had a vendetta against the blind people using Guide Horses, both from the perspective of a "guide dog only" preference and as miniature horse breeders.

People started publishing falsehoods about the program in online forums, suggesting that they were authorities on guide animal training techniques and on the needs and requirements of blind people like Dan Shaw. They posted that we charged money for the Guide Horses, and falsely claimed that the Guide Horse users must pay for their own training expenses. This was of course far from the truth as we always gave the horses free of cost to the handlers and we paid for all their training costs and equipment. Most of these expenses were paid out of our own funds as we did not have an active campaign to raise funds for the training program.

131

It was deeply offensive that someone would claim we were selling Guide horses thereby profiting from a program to which I was donating my time, services and personal funds so that the Guide horses could be free to the blind handlers. Unfortunately I was powerless to respond via the forum because I had been banned from the forum by the moderator even though I had never posted any messages there before. Noting that I was not responding to the misinformation, the posters became even bolder with the anti-Guide horse messages posted as well as messages demanding to know Dan Shaw and Shari's personal medical information so that they might judge if they were "blind enough" to use Guide animals.

Personalized Harassment

On the evening of June 8, 2004 we were hit with the worst assault ever directed against a Guide Horse user. Untrue details were published about Shari and her Guide Horse Tonto's Scout on an Internet forum. They went so far as to claim that Tonto only had two weeks of training before he went to Shari. When in reality he was in training for almost two years and we had spent four weeks training Shari to use her guide horse safely.

One post read that they knew where Shari lived and also suggested that stealing Tonto from Shari was the way to stop her from using a Guide horse.

Words could not express my fear after reading this. It was terrifying that someone knew where Shari lived and planned to interfere with her right to use the mobility aid of her choice. We had closely guarded her personal contact information, only saying with her permission that she lived in Pennsylvania but someone Shari had met in her hometown shared her address with the conspirators.

Shari's dilemma

Shari, being a private person, had always made it clear that she wanted to avoid controversy and publicity, preferring to use Tonto's Scout peacefully and without interference.

Dan Shaw had learned to deal with abuse from the small group of prejudiced people that tried to interfere with his right to use Cuddles as his guide animal. We were concerned that Shari would not be able to deal with this stress.

With that concern in mind Don called Shari and told her about this person's intent to contact her. When Don read her the published comments she was puzzled.

"It's untrue", she said. "I love Tonto and he is a good guide." She lamented " I cannot imagine why anyone would be hateful enough to say these things".

Shari's voice became very strained: *"Oh My God, what can I do?"* Shari said quietly. *" I can't live my life in constant fear"*.

Shari was distraught, immediately fearing for the safety of Tonto's Scout. We had not yet told her about the talks to seize him, but she guessed what was going to happen next. Shari decided to call and confront the person, hopefully before her home address was widely distributed.

Shari and her husband called me back later, saying that they telephoned the woman and informed her that she was spreading misinformation, asking her to stop publishing falsehoods and please leave them alone. I followed up with a letter to this woman, letting her know about the damage that she had caused and inviting her to take the time to learn more about the Guide Horse program before condemning the participants.

To everyone's surprise, she later admitted that she had published false information.

Thrilled that she had accepted responsibility, we remained hopeful that this would blow over and Shari could return to her peaceful existence. Sadly, that was not to be the case. This lady was on a crusade to prevent blind people from using the service animal of their choice. She was not finished with Shari, and continued to assert that Shari and Dan should not be allowed to use horses as guide animals.

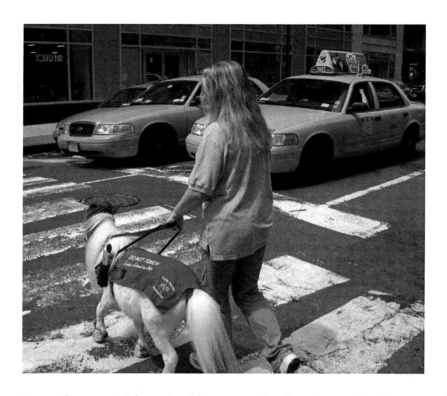

One of our neighbors had been monitoring the online forum and stopped over at our house to express her sorrow at the way Dan and Shari were being attacked. Penny is a miniature horse breeder who shares our outrage at the unjustified harassment of innocent blind people. Penny said that she could not go online to help defend us. She had tried to present the positive viewpoint on the forum before, only to find her messages removed by the moderators. So she knew that there was no way to respond to the threats in that venue. However, Penny had a revelation for us:

"I know her," she spoke of Shari's attacker.

"I saw her at a horse show just a few months ago competing in a cart competition. By her own admission she is totally blind.

"She didn't have her guide dog running out in front of her in that class and she relied on her horse to guide her around the show ring and the show grounds."

The next day brought a teary phone call from Shari telling me that she could not continue to live with the stress of the harassment. She reiterated that she loved Tonto's Scout very much and enjoyed working with him, but the threats and controversy were too much for her and her family to deal with. Out of love for her family and concern for their well being she made the decision to part with her beloved fuzzy pony.

Tonto's Scout returned home to the Guide Horse Foundation on June 18, 2004. Scout is an excellent horse and after a suitable retraining period he will hopefully have a chance to work with a new handler.

The crusade against Shari's right to choose her service animal was victorious. Prejudice had robbed her of the right to learn through experience if she and Tonto could be a successful Guide Horse team in the suburbs.

Donna 's Pal

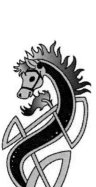

It was obvious from the first moment that Donna was an ideal candidate for a Guide Horse. Donna has a lifelong love of horses, and she had trained a horse to win a State championship. Donna is intelligent, stable, and a big plus, she had a large pasture where her Guide Horse could run and play when he was off duty.

Upon first meeting Donna at her preliminary evaluation I immediately liked her. She was assertive and there was no doubt in her mind that she wanted to try a Guide Horse. Donna has exceptional mobility skills and a can do attitude. Impressed with her potential we scheduled her to come

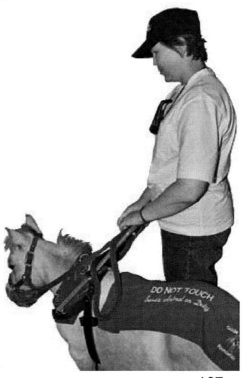

137

for three weeks of training in North Carolina.

Donna, a lifelong equestrian and champion western competition rider has won in barrels, poles, stake race, western riding and trail, all on the same horse, her beloved Rebel. Donna resides with her

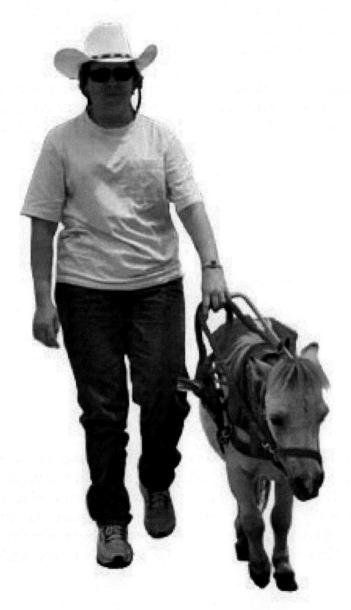

husband Tom in the heart of Texas. Donna and Rebel were the 1978 Texas State champions in youth pole bending. They competed in the Youth Quarter Horse World Finals for 3 years in a row, placing in the top ten their final year.

Donna and Rebel represented the State of Texas at the Quarter Horse Congress in Columbus, Ohio. They helped bring the Texas team to a 6th place finish, by placing in the top ten for barrels out of more than 100 riders.

A lifelong horse lover and accomplished horse trainer, Donna was a successful competitor even after losing her vision. Relying on Rebel to guide her, Donna learned to trust Rebel and continued to win competitions after her vision was impaired. Pole bending is an extremely challenging timed event where the horse and rider must navigate between a series of 6 poles, placed 21 feet apart and in a straight line. It is similar to a slalom skiing event. Sadly Rebel was killed by a lighting strike, and Donna has retired from competitive riding.

"I still miss him every day." Donna says, "He was such a large part of my life."

Donna now turns her considerable animal training experience to herding dog competitions where she has been very successful despite her blindness.

Donna passed her preliminary orientation and mobility skills assessment test in Spring 2003, and then later traveled to the Guide Horse Foundation for preliminary work with Pal, an exceptionally intelligent and friendly two year-old buckskin gelding, who weighed in at 125 pounds. Donna traveled to the Guide Horse Foundation in June 2003 where she performed preliminary guide work training and testing with Pal. Donna also took time out to do some riding while visiting North Carolina and successfully trotted and loped unassisted astride the 16 hand high chestnut gelding Raspberry Jam++, a champion National Show Horse and recipient of the prestigious Legion of Merit award.

Donna returned to the Guide Horse Foundation in November of 2003 for an intensive orientation and training where she learned to use Pal as her guide.

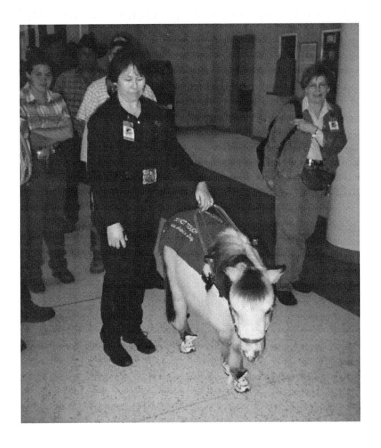

Pal was only two years old and twenty six inches high when he went home to work with Donna. Unfortunately Pal had not yet reached his mature height at that time. Expecting him to grow maybe another half an inch we were surprised that he grew another three inches over the next two years and gained thirty pounds! Suddenly the gentle horse was no longer small enough to perform properly as a Guide Horse.

Pal's large size became a barrier to his success as Donna's working partner. Working inside was awkward as he was too large to fit in many situations.

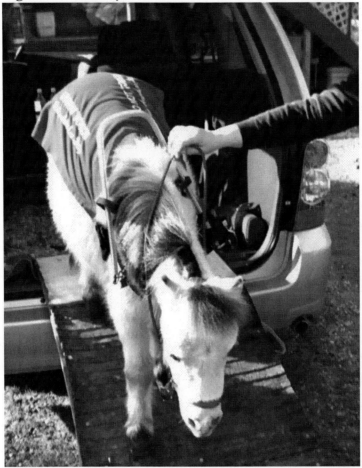

He couldn't fit in the family's vehicles. Traveling with Pal became so difficult that he and Donna were not able to work in public together on a regular basis. As Pal spent increasingly less time working and more time running free in his pasture his performance as a guide suffered.

As Donna continued having increasing problems with his performance we scheduled to bring Pal back to North Carolina.

There he would have a month of evaluation and a refresher course of guide training. Donna had developed a working bond as well as an attachment for Pal so we were reluctant to replace him if he could be reconditioned to perform in spite of the obstacles he now faced.

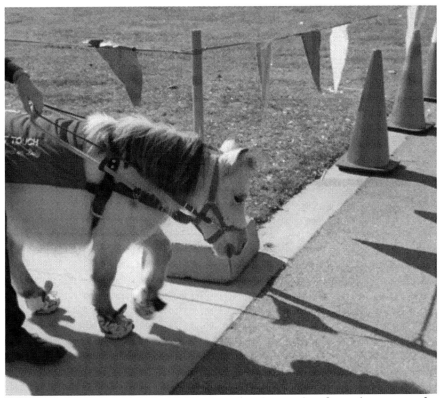

During the month that Pal spent back on the farm he seemed to settled in and show his original talent as we put him through his paces. But in spite of his willing and responsive attitude we noticed he had new physical hurdles to cross. Pal had developed stiffness in his shoulders and neck that restricted his flexibility while working. Attempts to retrain Pal seemed successful but as soon as he returned to his home environment it became obvious that he had a limited future as a working Guide horse.

Pal could no longer easily travel in the crucial shoulder-in position he had been trained to maintain while guiding. As Pal began to develop a habit of traveling in a straight forward position beside his handler he became less aware of the handler's needs in relation to the environment. Gradually he began to follow instead of lead. He was no longer effective as a Guide Horse.

No longer able to perform safely Pal was retired from working as a Guide Horse. Subsequently Pal returned to North Carolina to spend his days grazing in the pasture and running with his herd.

A great deal was learned from Donna and Pal's efforts during their time spent working together. Most important was the realization that while a horse may be sufficiently trained to perform as a guide by age two it should be allowed to fully mature physically before entering a working team relationship. In the future horses would not be placed as working guides until after their fifth birthday thus preventing problems caused by unexpected growth and conformation changes.

Donna and Pal also contributed to the study of traveling procedures and requirements for Guide Horses.

Travel Training

With the growing interest in using miniature horses as guides I was always on the lookout for opportunities to clear-up misconceptions and allow the Guide Horse users to tell others what their Guide Horse means to them.

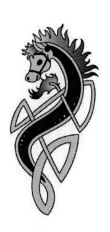

We received a call from the hit television show "ER" asking if we could provide a blind person and a Guide Horse for one of their upcoming episodes. As a great fan of the show I was very excited to contribute the services of a horse so that more people would be exposed to the concept. Of course we couldn't accept payment for the appearance but they agreed to cover our expenses giving us a chance to take a horse on a air flight training mission that we otherwise couldn't have afforded to do. The writer had read about Dan and Cuddles in Newsweek and had decided that Guide horses deserved a place in his series. I reviewed his script and was pleasantly surprised at the plot, deciding that an appearance on ER would be excellent exposure for working Guide horses.

We decided to use Scout for the filming after he won third-place in the World Championship miniature horse competition and because he was an excellent guide and extremely tiny. The first step was getting Scout on the airplane. He had never flown before so we enlisted the aid of Dan Shaw as an experienced Guide horse user that had flown a lot with his Guide horse Cuddles. Dan was happy to help out as he always enjoys helping train the new horses.

We have had an excellent relationship with Delta airlines, and they were thrilled to have Dan and Scout to take their first solo flight together. Scout performed wonderfully on the 6 hour flight and became a hit with the flight attendants. Delta trains their flight attendants about working with passengers with Guide horses, and the pilot personally welcomed Scout during his pre-flight announcement.

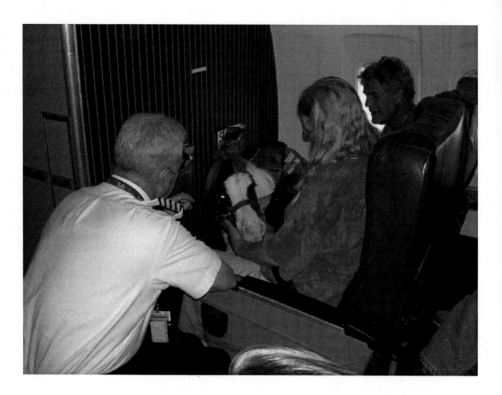

Upon arrival in California we settled into a Marriott hotel for the six days required to film the three complex scenes required by ER. When we checked Dan and Scout into their room I made sure that Dan understood Scouts "go" signals and how to get to the outdoor relief area. Because of the jet-lag, I also decided that we should but a diaper on Scout at night, just to be safe and save Dan from a middle-of-the-night trip through the hotel lobby.

The first morning I awoke to the chaos of getting to the studio for the 8:00 AM call. Dan called at 5:00 AM and announced that Scout was packing a full-load. Now, I know that Dan is a doting grandfather, so I knew that he understood how to change a diaper. *"Just pull off the diaper and bag it"*, I suggested. *"Whatever you do, don't flush the nuggets down the toilet"* Horse manure is very high fiber, and it doesn't flush well.

148

When we went by his room to pick up Dan and Scout laterthat morning Dan answered the door with a complaint. *"The Toilet overflows when I try to flush it"*. We had to call housekeeping, and discovered that Dan had not taken Scout outside on a late night relief break. Instead, Dan had flushed the high-fiber horse manure down the toilet.

When we arrived at Warner Bros. Studios we were giver the VIP treatment and enjoyed full access to the ER set. The ER show is incredibly complex and bustling with hundreds of supplemental actors, who work to provide a backdrop for the central characters. My first task was to desensitize Scout to the chaotic set and make sure that he understood his role in the episode.

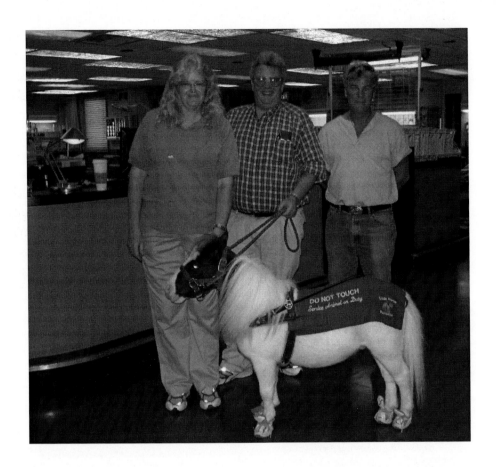

We were not aware that a 50 minute episode of ER required 8 full days of shooting, with each day often running more than ten hours. They explained that ER has earned 21 Emmy Awards and 108 nominations, breaking an all-time industry record, partially because of their attention to perfection and detail. The writer for ER was stickler for accuracy and detail and Dan Shaw was able to provide advice for Jane, the actress who was playing the blind Guide Horse user.

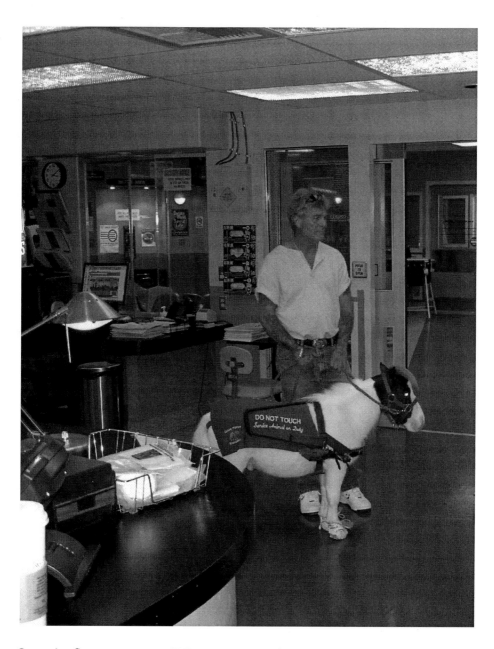

Scout's first scene on ER was a carefully choreographed long-shot where the main characters see the blind woman and her guide horse. With over 50 characters in the scene, timing was critical and Scout and the Blind woman had to walk and hit their "mark" at precisely the right moment. This required Scout to walk at exactly the same cadence between takes and I was thrilled when we were able to get the scene perfect after only 30 minutes. The stars of ER, Maura Tierney (Abby) and Noah Wyle (Dr. Carter) were very nice, and I was happy to hear that Noah was a miniature horse owner and very familiar with their intelligence and skill. *"I've got both big horses and mini's on my farm and I know how smart they are"*, Noah told me. *"It's a real pleasure to meet you, Scout"*.

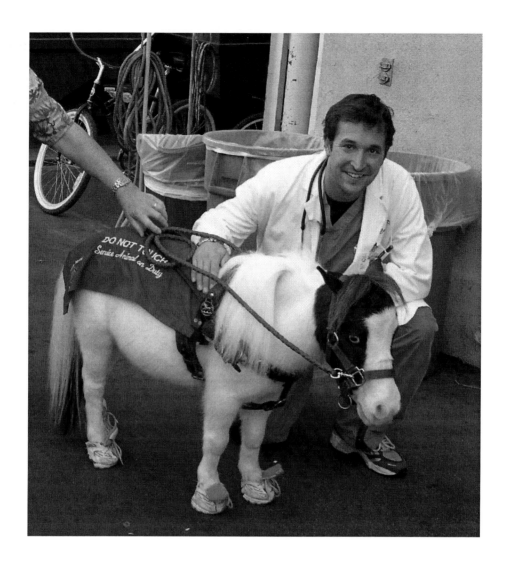

The shooting was very stressful, and the director seemed exasperated in getting the complete silence he needed from the 100+ people on the busy set. When we came in to shoot the first scene, the director tried to make us feel comfortable. *"This horse is going to be a big star"*, the director announced to the room: *"You had better treat him with respect since he could be the next Mr. Ed"*. The actors laughed, but it put even more pressure on me to make sure that I cued him properly.

The first scene required Don to release Scout and Jane on-cue, while I had to scramble 20 feet on my hands and knees backwards, just out of camera range. Don said that I looked like a land crab as I scooted backward 25 feet after the director cried *"Rolling ... Speed. ... Start background. ... Action!"*. On this cue, I released Scout and crawled backwards for 25 feet, all while keeping Scouts attention on me so he would know where to take Jane. The scene required Scout and Jane to appear at precisely the right moment and it required Scout to walk at exactly the same pace between takes. I was mortified when Scout walked too fast during the first take and missed his mark. *"Don't worry"*, one of the staffers said. *"It's not uncommon to have dozens of takes on every scene. The director is a perfectionist and it is demanding for everyone."*

Despite the chaos and my anxiety, subsequent takes went well, and I was thrilled to hear the director shout *"PERFECT ... Print! ... Great Job!"*. Now Scout had only three more scenes to go.

In the second scene Scout and the actress had to sit in the hall of the ER for an extended period while Abby and Dr. Carter discussed why Guide Horses should have full access to hospitals. During this scene Abby and Carter justify to a clerk about why "Ruby" (Scout's stage name) was allowed to stay in the ER. *"He can stay"*, Dr. Carter said and the director shouted "CUT! Ruby is a girl pony". *"Sorry"*, Noah said *"I know that Scout is a boy and I got confused!"*.

Scout stood perfectly still and muzzled Dr. Carter when he petted him, making for an irresistible scene. The producers and directors were thrilled with Scout's premier performance and we received many complements from the actors and staff about Scout.

154

The next two scenes were far more challenging. In the shoot, Scout was required to look-up with concern at Jane while Abby treated an injury to her hand. Following this take, Scout was required to reach up and sympathetically lick the wound on the back of Jane's hand. After witnessing several days of shooting I was very nervous because of the high demands by the director for perfection. I had nightmares of Scout failing to walk over to the actress, failing to lick her hand, or worse yet, grabbing her hand and biting her!

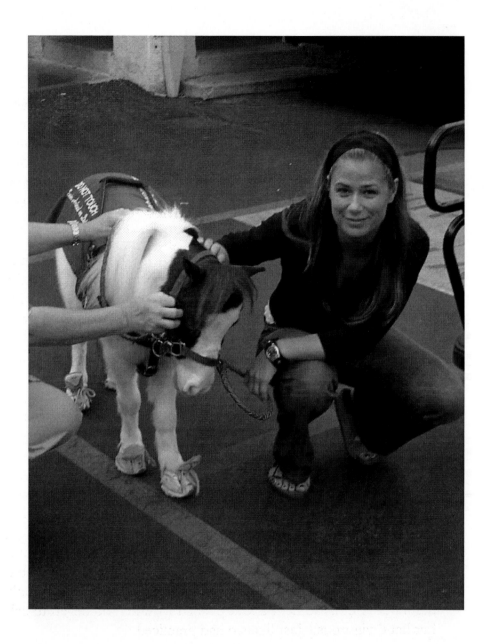

There was a great deal of concern about the licking requirement because licking is not a natural behavior for a horse, plus as a Guide Horse Scout had been taught to not put his mouth on a human at any time. What if the filming was delayed if Scout was not able to immediately lick Jane's hand?

It took several days of rehearsal to get the scene outline just right, and one of the biggest problems was Scout's small size. At only 26 inches, tall, Scout was too small to reach-up to Jane's hand, and a special cut-down medical tray had to be customized so that Scout could reach her hand. This cut-down tray meant that Maura (Abby) had to squat-down on a super short stool, but she took the challenge with great goodwill.

When we entered to film the scene, there was a funny little miniature stuffed horse that was being used as a stand-in for the preliminary shooting. I stopped Scout by the stuffed toy to give him a chance to examine it so he could understand that it was nothing to worry about. Curious he sniffed it all-over, trying to understand if it might be a new friend. *"Where is Scout Now?"* the director shouted.

"E's over 'ere sniffing the stand-in's bum" a crew member with a heavy cockney accent shouted, and the whole set laughed.

Stepping up the pace we took our place next to Abby, and I directed Scout to try to reach-up into the tray table. Scout complied by resting his entire head on the table, and gazing up at Abby as if to say *"OK, here I am"*. *"Oh my God, that's the cutest thing I've ever seen"* Abby laughed, and I pulled Scout's head down and signaled him to lick the fake wound without putting his whole head on the tray! He hesitated to touch the unfamiliar person's hand but after a moment Scout pushed forward and began to lick her hand vigorously just like we had practiced.

Finally, the ER shooting was completed and it was time to get back to work training Scout to work properly as a guide.

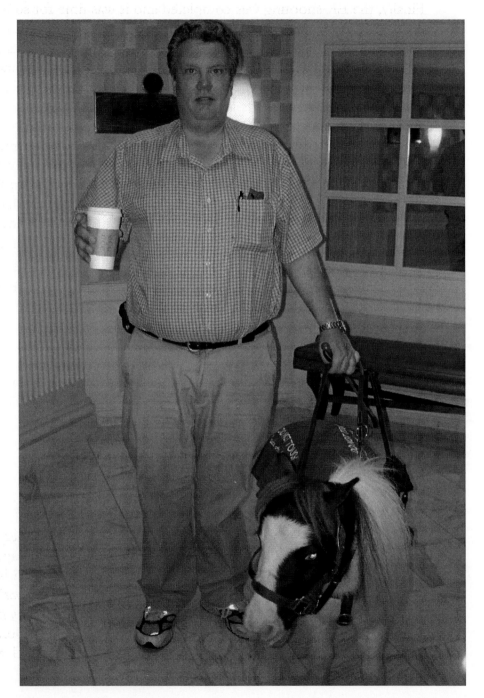

Finally, the ER shooting was completed and it was time for some serious training. Donna and Pal flew up from Texas to join us so they could get in some travel experience also. Given the basic differences in traveling with a horse we wanted to invest the time and effort to attempt to cover all the bases and help the horses learn to be good travel companions.

After Donna and Pal arrived, we went everywhere, even sitting in the studio audience for the Jay Leno "Tonight Show". Donna was adamant that she did not want any special recognition. During the warm-up Jay Leno could not help but notice that there were two horses in his studio audience. The Tonight Show staff wanted to acknowledge our presence and the staff had a quick meeting. Always politically correct, they decided that it might be offensive to point-out people just because they used a unique guide animal. *"That's a load off my mind"*, Donna said. *"I just want to see the show"*.

Everywhere we wandered; people were friendly and excited that Guide horses had finally appeared in California. Donna remarked about how helpful and supportive the California people were and now she was welcomed everywhere that she went.

Getting Along Together

Now, Donna and Don are very different people and I was very concerned about their being able to get-along during our 10 days together. For example, Don is a chain smoker while Donna is severely allergic to cigarette smoke. *"Put that horrible thing out"* Donna shouted at Don from across the parking lot. *"Yeesh, I must be 20 feet away from you, how can you possibly small my smoke?"* Don replied. On the 90 minute drive back to the Burbank hotel a radio commercial blared *"Every day Californians are killed by second-hand smoke. . . . Don't let these people kill you"*.

One day we walked to the elevator and smelled the pungent odor of marijuana in the hallway. "Christ, you can smoke a joint in this state but heaven help you if you light a cigarette" Don noted. "This state is very different than North Carolina. You can't even smoke on the beach".

Somehow we worked it out, and despite the stress of navigating the LA freeways and chaos, everyone got along as well as could be expected. One afternoon we decided to drive out to Malibu to gawk at the hillside mansions and eat in Wolfgang Puck's premier restaurant "Granita".

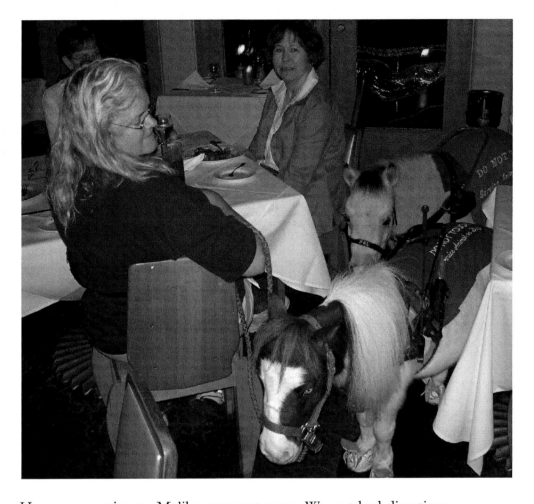

However, getting to Malibu was not easy. We got bad directions from the hotel and we were soon in the clutches of horrendous LS freeway gridlock. Since Don could not smoke with Donna in the van, things got tense real *fast* *"Jeez, I HATE this F****** traffic"* Don screamed after the first 30 minutes of stop-and-go. About this time Scout started signaling that he had to pee and we were at least 20 minutes from the next freeway exit. At this point, both Scout and Don were very irritable and Don took the first exit, stopping at a gas station. Don grabbed Scout and stood there on a small patch of grass, Scout whizzing and Don puffing away.

Nearly two hours after starting out, we finally arrived in Malibu and pulled into the mall parking lot just before dark. Weaving between the Ferrari's and Rolls Royce's, Scout and Pal did an excellent job in Malibu and we were warmly greeted by the locals. One upscale woman, sporting a solid gold Rolex encrusted with diamonds approached us, asking the usual questions and chuckling out-loud when we said that we were there to grace Granita with our presence.

Ever since Dan and Cuddles went to the Palm Court restaurant in New York City for afternoon tea, we have always enjoyed taking Guide horses into upscale restaurants. The look on the server's faces is priceless, and you can almost hear there brains racing as they try to figure out how to handle their most unusual guests. We were treated warmly and seated in a back corner of Granita, where we tucked Scout and Pal under the table. Nobody noticed that we has horses until halfway through the meal Pal sneezed, making an unmistakable horse-like noise that made everyone look around the dining area. Always the clown, Don pulled a handkerchief from his pocket and pretended that he had sneezed like a horse.

Hollywood

After the filming we visited Hollywood and Beverly Hills, playing tourist and visiting Grauman's Chinese Theatre, walking Hollywood Boulevard amidst the crowds of tourists.

162

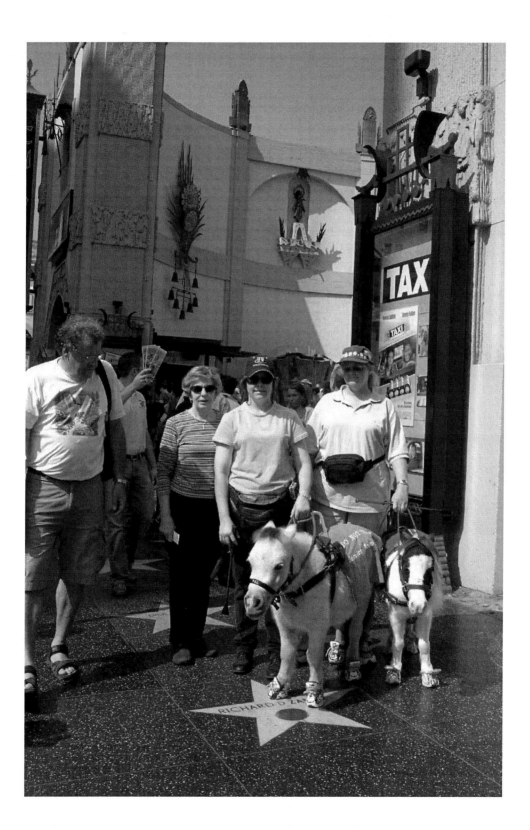

Now, Hollywood Boulevard is not as upscale as it was in its heyday, and we were surprised to see several scary people walking the streets. Many appeared to be on mind-altering drugs and I especially questioned the sanity of one scraggly couple of punkers. They wore brightly-colored spiked hair, body piercing of every visible appendage (and some no visible, I'm sure), jackets replete with metal and spikes and most amazing of all, they were bonded together with a chain running between their pierced cheeks!

Even Scout briefly looked-up at the remarkable couple with neon green and blue hair while I wondered about the damage that they would suffer if one of them tripped and fell!

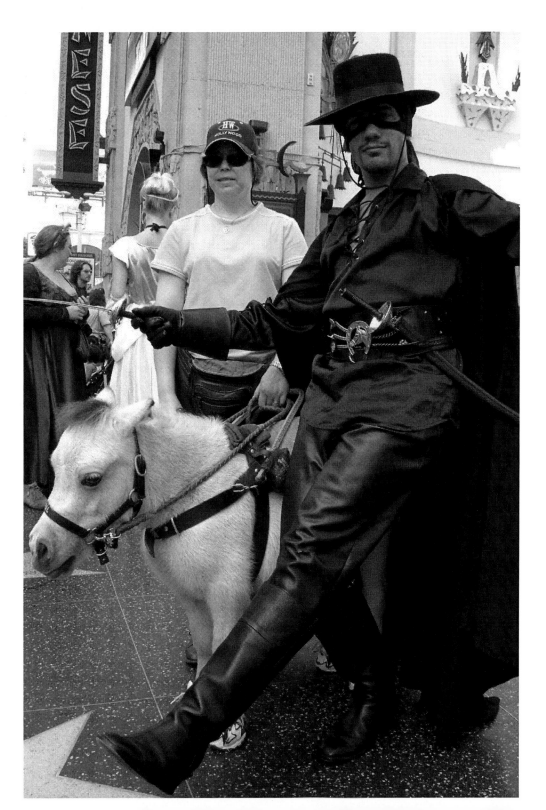

Amidst the teaming hordes of tourists we encountered a great real-world training area. At one intersection a pedestrian stepped directly in front of Pal as he led Donna across a busy intersection. Donna could hear the obstruction and ordered "FORWARD". Pal seemed to know exactly what was going on and proceeded ahead navigating around the obstruction.

You would think that in the land of "anything goes", the natives would be tolerant of the unusual, but that was not always the case. With decades of "Hollywood Schmaltz" and endless publicity stunts, many natives are naturally suspicious of anything unusual. *"Ha, that the funniest thang I ever done seen",* one wino said to Dan as he walked down Hollywood Boulevard. *"What's so funny about being blind?"* Dan shot back, obviously perturbed at the bum's insensitive remark. Once the hobo realized that Dan was the real-deal, he looked very embarrassed and slunk back into the alley.

Deciding it was time to move to a more upscale neighborhood we drove to Beverly Hills. We walked up-and-down Rodeo drive and dined in a fancy restaurant with a sidewalk café, replete with upscale people and their tiny dogs, some eating directly from their master plates. Now this may be anthropomorphism, but it seemed to me that with Pal and Scout and we were especially amused to see the misbehavior of these spoiled pets, casting a gaze in their direction as we enter the fancy eatery. Relaxing after working hard, Pal and Scout slept quietly while we ate. *"Would you like a seat outside?"* the tuxedoed Matre'de pleaded in a poor French accent, obviously unhappy at the prospect of having livestock in his restaurant. *"No, there are too many naughty dogs out there",* Donna replied and the stuffy faux monsieur shrugged and guided us to an inside table.

166

Las Vegas

That weekend we piled into the mini-van and set-out on the 4-hour drive to Las Vegas. We were visiting Las Vegas to give a presentation to the Las Vegas Blind Services department and to see how the Guide horses would work in the chaos of a crowded casino. During the long drive through the desolate desert, Don puffed on his fat cigars while Scout and Pal snacked on hay and watched the scenery out the back on the minivan.

Within minutes of checking in to the MGM Grand, we were greeted by an army of uniformed security guards at our hotel room door. *"Excuse me"*, an obviously embarrassed guard said. *"This is going to sound really bizarre, but the man monitoring the security cameras said that two horses entered the hotel, rode the elevator and walked into your rooms."* At this point I was tempted to have some fun with the guards but I decided to play it straight. *"Yes, we have horses in our rooms"*, I replied, opening the door to reveal Pal and Scout, who stopped exploring their rooms and looked over at the amazed guards with a quizzical gaze. *"They are Guide horses. You've seen Guide horses before haven't you?"*, I said.

"Um, Yeah, of course we have", the Sergeant replied. "We just needed to confirm it."

I showed them Pal and Scouts certification cards and politely reminded them that disabled people are not required to produce papers everywhere they travel. *"Oh yes, we know"* the contrite Sergeant said. *"You've been really nice, and we appreciate it. I'll make a note for Security in all the nearby hotels to make sure that nobody challenges you. If they do, just say ADA, and they will leave you alone"*. We thanked the Sergeant and his entourage and they radioed to the security room that Guide horses were staying as guests.

Later that day I got a call from the head of hotel safety asking questions. *"We get lots of guide dogs here"*, he said, "but you are the first Guide horses to stay at the MGM". *With guide dogs owners we have to ask for certificates of worming because dogs might carry parasites that can pass to humans. I was happy to find that horses don't carry parasites that can transmit diseases to people, and that makes my job a whole lot easier. Plus, I won't have to have the rooms disinfected".* This poor man was obvious concerned about safety, so I spent a few minutes with him explaining that horses are generally non-allergic, normally do not host fleas, and have no known transmittable diseased to humans. I also offered to give him copies of Pal's and Scout's health certificates to ease his mind.

Donna had not been to Las Vegas in several years and she was anxious to strike-out on her own. While seeking-out the slot machines, Donna and Pal were accustomed to answering questions from passerby's. Always polite, Donna always takes time to talk with everyone. One fellow came up to Donna with dozens of questions, and after hearing her answers, expressed great approval. Once he left, another passerby approached Donna *"Do you know who you were taking with? That was Howie Mandell, the comedian who is headlining at the MGM. What did you say to him?"*

"Well" Donna replied, *"I just answered his questions and asked him where the quarter slots were. He was very helpful!"*

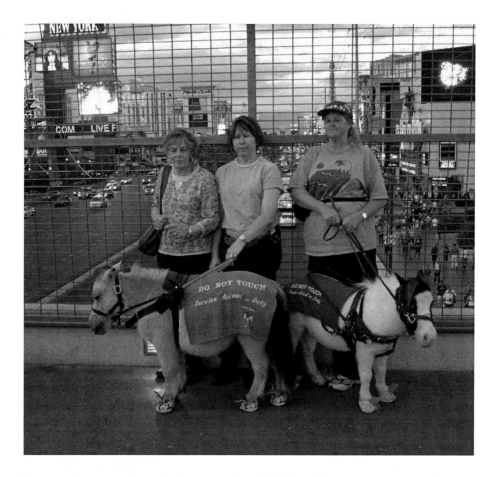

Donna then approached me and said "I really want to go to the Howie Mandell show tonight. He's was really nice and he supports us, so we should support him back". Not wanting to disappoint Donna by mentioning how hard it is to get tickets on the day of the show, I politely agreed and set-out to find a way to get seats for four people and two horses for the evening show. Fortunately, the Concierge at the MGM was extremely helpful and we got center-stage seats. We had a great time at the show, and all of us laughed until we cried.

During this time I wanted to see how Scout handled the chaos on a busy casino floor and the hoards on Las Vegas Strip, so I enlisted Don to help. The MGM Grand was full of people from all over the world, and we really enjoyed the cosmopolitan atmosphere of the hotel.

One day while Don and Donna were in the lobby with Pal and Scout a Japanese woman approached Donna repeating *"For Pony, For Pony"*, and stuffed a dollar bill into Donna's hand! After I verified the denomination of the bill, Donna replied *"I should have told her that we only take hundreds!"* The woman's gift bought a small bag of mints for Pal, and Pal thoroughly enjoyed them.

Pal is the only horse that I have ever seen who enjoys sucking on mints. When Pal gets a cherished mint he sticks his neck out, half closes his eyes and makes an audible slurping noise for more than five minutes. While standing in the lobby, several guests were flabbergasted at seeing a Guide Horse in sneakers, standing quietly by the gaming table having a mint-induced horse organism. *"Man, he's sure likes his treat"* a lady said. *"How long does he do that?"* *"I timed him at 12 minutes last night"* Donna chuckled, happy to see that even non-horse owners found Pal's profound enjoyment to be hilarious.

"Animals are such beautiful creatures", one woman commented while Scout took a nap at the blackjack table. While I pondered than meaning of this comment, a gambler rushed over from the craps table and asked if he could pet Scout for luck. I agreed, and the man did a quick pat and retuned to his table, full of confidence. Several minutes later I heard a huge scream coming from the table. *"I just won $12,000"*, the man said, panting and visibly excited.*" This is truly a remarkable pony. Thank you."* I smiled and

returned to my game. Privately, I wondered if I should pet Scout more often, since I had lost five hands in a row! Even though she is blind, Donna loved playing blackjack, and everyone at the table was telling her the "up" cards and giving her suggestions.

Our visit with the Las Vegas Blind Services staff went well, and several blind people and Orientation and Mobility instructors took a Juno walk with Scout to understand the subtle differences between Guide horse and guide dogs. During the presentation I explained the benefits and drawbacks of using a Guide horse and I was sure to explain that Guide horses did not compete with guide dogs.

During our presentation Pal signaled Donna that he had to "go" and the whole room followed us outside to see Pal relieve himself! Donna had kept Pal in extremely excellent training, and he immediately stretched out and emptied his bladder. "I'm really impressed", one staffer said. *"Many of the guide dogs have accidents, especially in strange surroundings".*

On the day of our departure, we all piled into the rented minivan, four people, two horses and 12 pieces of luggage. Upon unloading at the airport I felt like I was performing the old circus act where a dozen people emerge from a Volkswagen, all for the amazement of the skycaps at the curb! Our flight home was uneventful, even though Scout was not an old-hand at flying.

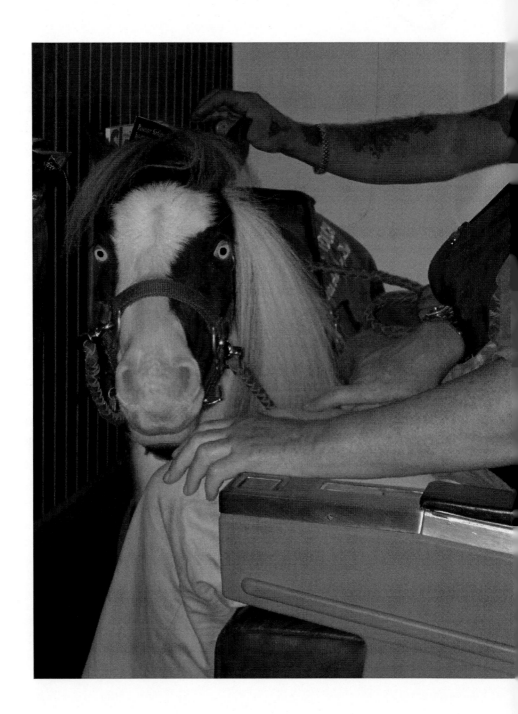

172

I found it interesting that when I finally released Scout back into the pasture with the herd at home at the end of his eleven day journey he immediately went up to Traveller, another Guide Horse in-training. Touching noses and snorting softly it was if Scout was telling Traveller about his great adventure flying to the West Coast.

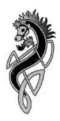

The West Coast trip presented a tremendous opportunity to explore the joys and trials of traveling with a Guide horse. During the course of the journey we learned many ways to care for the horses on the road, as well as learning that there was a lot more training ahead if the horses were to blend smoothly with a traveling lifestyle.

Confetti & Cheryl

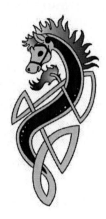

Cheryl Spencer with her husband Chris visited us in 2001 meeting with us along with Dan Shaw with Cuddles. She tried out one of the horses we were currently training and decided she wanted a Guide horse. Unfortunately we didn't have enough horses to go around. Or enough hours in the day to train enough horses.

Long-time horse lovers, Cheryl and her husband Chris were saddened by our long waiting list and decided to pursue an owner trained guide, a right guaranteed by the Americans with Disabilities Act.

Cheryl tells people that she wanted a reliable long living replacement for her aging Seeing Eye dog "Delta", who passed away at the age of twelve recently after nearly a decade of faithful service.

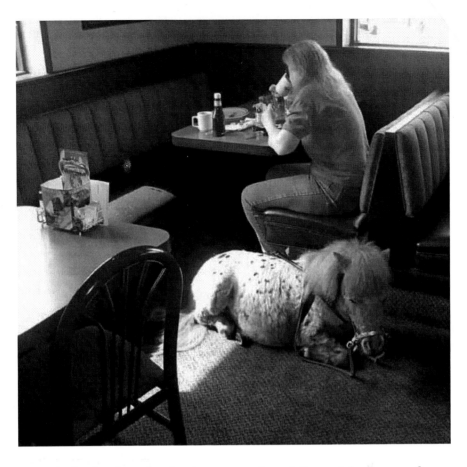

Cheryl obtained enthusiastic approval and financial support from her state Council for the Blind and was given charitable funding to acquire Confetti and the services of a professional horse trainer to assist Chris and Cheryl in their training endeavors. Confetti has been reported to be doing an exceptional job in keeping Cheryl safe despite her total blindness and has recently earned her wings, taking a grueling commercial flight.

"Confetti has earned her wings! We flew to Boston, MA, last weekend on Delta Airlines for my youngest daughter's high school graduation. Confetti flew in the cabin with us and stood in the bulkhead seat area."

Cheryl has reported great success in housebreaking Confetti, but like all responsible guide animal owners, they were fully prepared for any eventuality:

"Confetti did really well--better than I thought she would, and much better than Cheryl thought she would. We developed a poo bag system for her in anticipation of her being frightened having an accident on the plane. She surprised us both by not having an accident. She has become adept at emptying herself out when we are going in somewhere and holding it until we get back to the van.

We took her to pee in Atlanta, but she wasn't ready to poo there. She held it until we got into Logan, and finally couldn't hold it any longer. It was 5-1/2 hours from the time we left the van in Jacksonville and the time she let go in Logan. The poo bag system worked perfectly, and everything went into the bag. I took it off, tied it and gave it to a nearby cleaning person who gratefully disposed of it. No muss, no fuss, and, most importantly, no embarrassment!"

Their first-time flying experience was very similar to the experience of the horses we trained on their first commercial flights:

"On the plane, the first takeoff was a bit scary for her, but she handled it very well. The first landing also startled her a bit when the wheels touched down, but she is an amazingly adaptable little girl, and she took her cues from us. I talked soothingly to her on takeoff and landing, and that seemed to help her handle it.

The second takeoff was both easier and a bit scarier for her because she knew what was coming. But instead of spooking, she leaned against the bulkhead to brace herself! The second landing was no big deal at all. This time she leaned against us, and, of course, we were bracing for the engine reversal. She took it all in stride!"

Cheryl and Chris also reported that Confetti was quite adept at traveling in a rented vehicle, and adapted quite well to foreign surroundings:

"By the time we returned that minivan, she was a pro! She really showed us how much she both loves and trusts us and how much she enjoys being a guide. Speaking of which, Confetti was a tremendous help guiding Cheryl

176

through the airports while I dealt with the luggage.. . . She is an amazing little girl!"

Cheryl reports that Confetti has bladder control on-par with her previous Seeing Eye dog and has able to "hold it" for eleven hours:

"I can go on and on and on about her, but let me end by saying that the return trip was 11 hours, and she waited until we were in the parking lot in Jacksonville before she unloaded. She didn't wait to get to the van, but she tried. I forgot which parking lot I had parked in, and we ended up in the wrong one. While I was trying to find the van, Confetti enjoyed a salad we got for her in Atlanta."

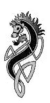

The experience of Cheryl and Confetti has confirmed what the experiment has indicated, that a blind person with the assistance and guidance of a professional horse trainer can train a guide horse to a suitable level. It will be interesting to follow Cheryl and Confetti over the next two decades to see how they continue to improve.

" I love your new shoes!"

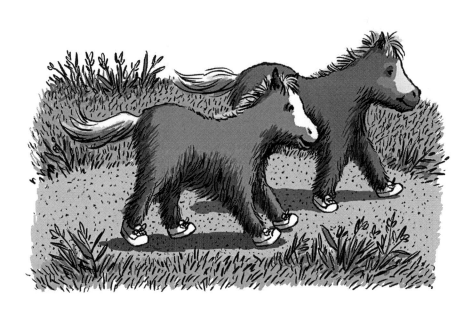

Traveler

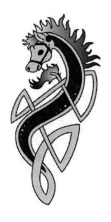

Penny, a wonderful lady and a trusted volunteer for the Guide Horse Foundation, had just found a group of seriously neglected and dying miniature horses whose drunken owner was not caring for them. Concerned for their lives, Penny had devised a plan where we might be able to convince the owner that it was in their best interests to allow us to restore them to health. Penny described a heart-wrenching situation of suffering, abuse and neglect, and I knew we had to act fast.

However Penny has some cautionary words - - *"If we bring Don, he's got to promise to keep his mouth shut"* said Penny. *"I know how he is about abused horses, and he needs to hold-his-tongue if we are going to save these ponies".*

We drove through the backwoods for over an hour before arriving at a dilapidated single-wide house trailer and some wooden shacks that reminded me of the National Geographic shows about third-world countries. Standing in the yard we saw the reason for our mission – a group of neglected and starving miniature horses, two stallions, five mares and several emaciated foals. I had made-up my mind that I was going to do whatever it took to save these sad animals.

Their owner, who was obviously drunk and stinking of alcohol, invited us into his trailer, and the sour smell of stale beer, vomit and urine hit us in the face. Penny had warned us about this former used-car salesman and Christian preacher who had kept his wife's' miniature horses after she had abandoned him, in hopes of using them as leverage during his divorce.

Choking-back the nauseating smell, we engaged this smelly disheveled drunkard in a discussion about his mini horses. According to Penny, he needed money fast (for liquor, no doubt) and was interested in selling the whole herd. He also had read stories about me the Guide Horse Foundation and knew that I was an animal lover.

When we inspected the miniature horses we did our best to control our outrage. They had virtually no food except for inedible moldy-hay and a stagnant water source that was polluted with feces and green algae. Several of the horses were deathly-ill and in-need of immediate medical attention, all of them lethargic and suffering, but the drunkard seemed oblivious to all of the suffering going-on all around him.

Most sad of all were Traveler, Hidalgo and Comanche, a stallion and two foals that were penned in a dark pen, a foot-deep in feces, where they were being neglected and starved. Hips bulging, you could count their ribs at 30 paces. As I choked-back

182

tears, it was clear that these poor creatures were his prisoners and I was determined to save them if I could.

Sadly, this was not the first time I had witnessed this wholesale abuse of innocent miniature horses. The glut of miniature horses caused by personal greed and the promise of quick riches (a top-quality miniature horse can fetch more than $30,000 at auction) has caused a serious problem. Profit-motivated poor people are buying breeding stock in record numbers and recklessly creating miniature horses in hopes of cashing-in on a big payday.

With prices for pet-quality miniature horses dropping down to their meat value (ten cents per pound), many poverty-stricken were buying them from killer auctions for less than $100 each and starting their own backyard breeding programs. I sometime wonder what is worse, being bled-to death in a slaughterhouse for a Frenchman's dinner, or being kept by breeders to treat them like livestock.

Often as not these tiny victims suffer and die if they became ill, primarily because of their owner's inability to provide them with proper veterinary care. My vet, Dr. Chris O'Malley told us of stories where a miniature horse owner had their horse euthanized rather than pay $200 for a life-saving medical procedure. I thought of the saying "being treated like cattle", and I was reminded that horse are livestock and not subject to the same humane treatment laws as dogs and cats.

Dealing with the Devil

As a preacher and used-car salesman, this obnoxious drunkard slurred his way through a sales pitch, oblivious to the dire needs of his tiny charges. "I wants fifteen hundred dollars each" he shouted and my heart sank. I knew that some of his ponies would be dead within a week if we did not get them medical attention.

Penny suspected that he was an alcoholic and he was running out of beer money. Boldly, she proposed a deal where we would buy his whole herd. The preacher's next statement was shocking – "Wall, what am I gonna to do for breeding if I sell my mares?" he said.

That's when Don could no-longer control his anger. "You have no business having horses that you can't afford to take care of, much less making more babies", Don said. At this point, Penny shrugged, regretting inviting Don and knowing that the negotiations were now in jeopardy.

"Wall, it's not my fault" explained the drunk, launching into a long tale-of-woe about how his wife had taken all his money and left him high-and-dry. Like many of the addicts I had read about in college psychology classes, this man believed that his own shortcomings were not his fault. We sat there for over 20-minutes, trying to be polite, listening to how none of this was his fault. My eyes began to water from the sour stench of the trailer.

"You have a lot of nerve sayin bad things about me in my own home", he finally said to Don, and I knew that if I did not intercede a fight was imminent. I scanned the room for guns and felt hard knot in my stomach.

Don has never been one to mince words, and he launched into his own tirade – "You sir, are detestable and I hope you rot in Hell", Don said as he left the stinking trailer to wait in the car. With the conflict avoided, and relaxed and I secretly I envied Don for finding an excuse to breathe some fresh air.

184

Playing the role of "good cop" Penny and I tried to finagle a deal where we might saves the lives of these innocent victims. I choked-back my own disgust when the drunk announced "I can't take a cent less than twenty five hundred dollars for the whole herd. These is valuable horses and I can't afford to give 'em away".

We politely thanked him and said we would think about it, leaving the dilapidated stink-hole for the clean air of the countryside. As we drove away I choked-back tears I saw the poor mini horses fade into the distance, and was appalled at this bold and uncaring attitude. The drunken preacher knew about my love and respect for animals and I saw his demand for top-dollar as nothing more than blatant extortion, with the pony's lives being used as leverage.

Out of the ten neglected horses there were only two that were suitable as Guide Horses, Traveler, the neglected stallion and Hidalgo the starving foal. Penny said that she could find homes for the other horses but we still had the issue of money.

Every year I spend thousands of dollars of my personal funds on food and medical care for neglected miniature horses, but twenty five hundred dollars was exorbitant by any measure. Most people will gladly give me their starving, crippled or neglected horses, usually, I suspect, to ease their guilty conscience.

As I sat there pondering this sad situation, Penny offered to kick-in some of her personal money. "I knew it was a bad idea to bring Don", she said, bringing a little levity to a desperate situation. "The last thing he needed to hear was the truth", and we all laughed.

"I've dealt with these dirt bag mini breeders before, and money talks. Let's come back tomorrow with 20 hundred dollar bills. I'll chip-in twelve hundred of my own money, and maybe we can save these horses, but I've got to do this alone" Penny said. I agreed to chip-in eight hundred dollars of my own money, and the next day Penny was able to secure the starving herd.

On Death and Dying

After scrambling to remove the horses, Penny conducted triage and concluded that lots of TLC, wormer and a nourishing diet would save most of the horses. Penny recalled the deal to me: "He wasn't happy at only two thousand dollars, but I've never seen an alcoholic yet how wouldn't pass on easy drinking money. By the way, he said that he did not want any of the horses to go to that Bastard Don". Don and I laughed, thrilled that we had saved the horses. "I'll be a bastard any day of the week if it means saving starving horses" Don said.

However, we were soon to learn about the real extent of the abuse. Blood work was done on Hidalgo, and Dr. O'Malley said that the poor baby was eating worm-infested feces to survive, riddling his intestines with parasites. "He was weaned too early, and he need to go to the hospital now", Dr. O'Malley said, and I cracked open my checkbook.

Three days later we received the sad news. *"I could not save Hidalgo", Dr. O'Malley said. "I killed the worms, but his intestines were so badly damaged that he could not absorb any nutrition from his food. I've never seen a red cell count so low. I kept him on pain medication and Hidalgo died peacefully in his sleep last night".*

186

After I stopped crying, I allowed Dr. O'Malley to perform a necropsy on Hidalgo to document the preacher's abuse. The medical report was conclusive that Hidalgo had suffered and died as the result of neglect and we were incensed.

"It's bad enough that we had to pay top-dollar to save these horses, but we can't just allow this evil man to go unpunished".

Don does not suffer fools gladly, especially when lives are at-stake, and his hatred for this man was apparent. "I considered sending him a case of whiskey in the hopes that he drinks himself to death, but that's too good for him. Let's let the world know what he has done".

I had to agree with Don. After years of witnessing the horrors of horse neglect I was tired of turning the other cheek. Innocent horses were suffering and dying every day, and I feel powerless to stop it. Legally, horses are considered livestock, and they do not have the same legal rights as companion animals such as dogs and cats.

Slowly recovering from the loss of Hidalgo, I tortured myself wondering if I could have saved him if I had paid the $2,500 right away instead of waiting another day. Dr. O'Malley eased my conscience, telling me that one day would not have made a difference.

Saving the Herd

With Hidalgo gone forever, we turned our attention to the surviving horses. Penny and I worked hard to nurse them back to health, and we were trying to find something good that might come from this horror.

I was thrilled when Dan Shaw, the first Guide Horse user, volunteered to take Comanche, an emaciated foal to Maine. A real animal lover, Dan enlisted a friend and drove thousands of miles to North Carolina to pick-up the foal.

Dan took great pride in providing him with the care and attention he so desperately needed, and I'm happy to report that Comanche is now gaining weight and growing at a normal level. I'm so proud of Dan for helping this tiny victim, despite his own blindness.

To date, all of the remaining horses survive a testament to the wonderful work done by Penny, Dan and other volunteers.

I'm a Little Traveler

One of the rescued horses I kept was named "I'm a Little Traveler", a 13 year-old malnourished stallion that was very grateful to have a new lease on life. Bright, friendly and intelligent, Traveler possessed all of the qualities of a Guide Horse, and I decided to give him a chance to have a fulfilling life.

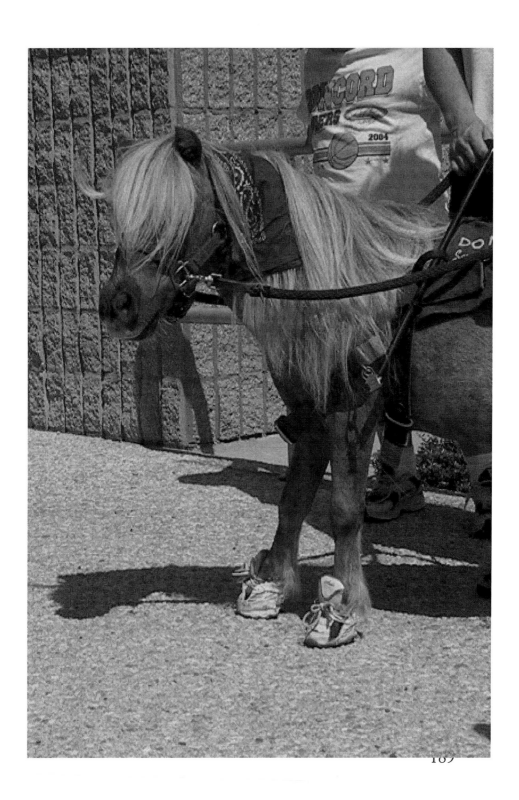

We had Traveler gelded, repaired his neglected hooves and placed him on a health regimen hoping that, unlike Hidalgo, the intestinal damage was not too great. Traveler thrived on the care and attention, gaining weight and muscle mass.

In my experience it can be very difficult to have an abused horse regain trust in humans and I was thrilled when Traveler became convinced that not all humans were evil and began to trust us.

The Training Begins

When training Traveler I was thrilled to discover that he was a "natural" for guide work. Having lived for years in a pit of his own feces, Traveler understood cleanliness and he was very easy to housebreak.

190

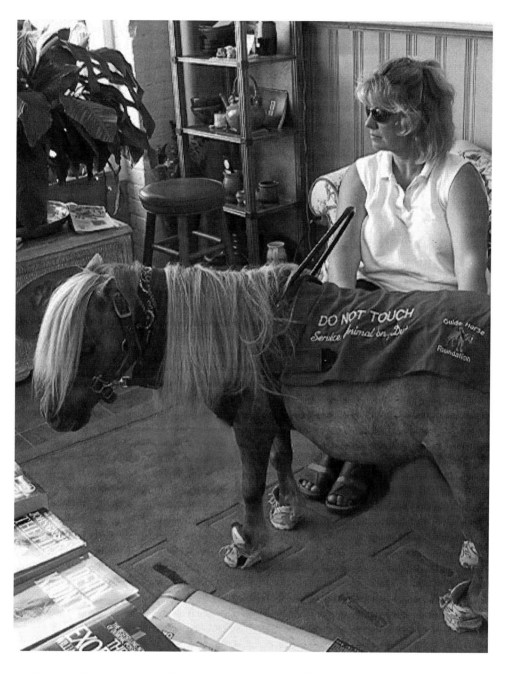

So far, Traveler has done a great job in his guide training. He is
still suspicious of humans that he does not know (a result of his

abuse, I suspect), but he has done very well in his basic guide training.

Full of wonder, I love taking Traveler out in public and I can sense his amazement at the new things he sees. The produce section of the supermarket was fascinating to Traveler and I wish that I could have captured the expression on his face.

When training Traveler, I always let him take some extra time to study new things. Once he got-over his natural fears and learned to trust me, I chuckle inside every time Traveler freezes in amazement at a new, wondrous object such as electronic doors or an escalator. I can only imaging how he must feel to see these things after years of confinement in a dark stall.

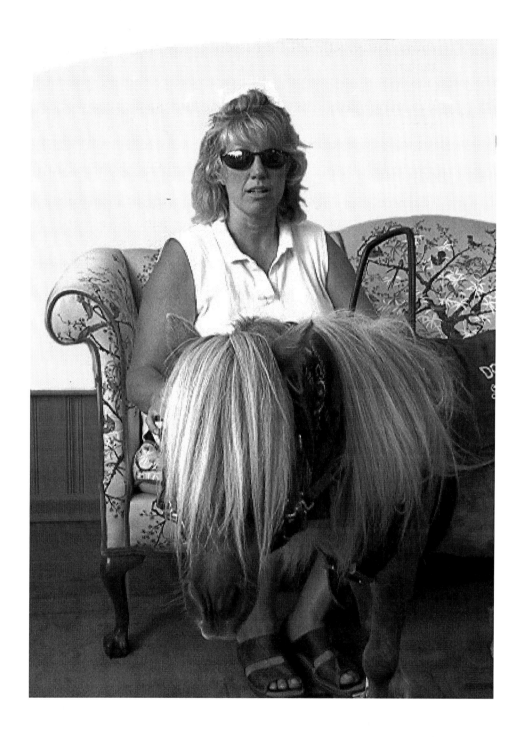

Today Traveler is coming along nicely and should be ready to place with a blind handler sometime soon. While all the Guide horses are special and we develop a special relationship with each of them, I feel especially close to Traveler because of his obvious gratitude and great personality.

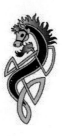

Service & Therapy

 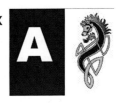
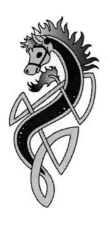

My husband Don has a degree in Psychology and worked for several years in an animal learning lab. He told me that Animal Psychologists choose a species based on the animal's natural predisposition to react in a certain way. For example, the super-sensitive ears of the Terriers make them ideal as hearing ear dogs. We had proof of this already because Chester (our Cairn terrier) reacts violently to loud noises and has been answering our telephone for years. If we don't Answer the phone fast, Chester leaps up and takes the receiver off the hook, growling and snarling at the caller. Once, after taking a long shower, I emerged to find the phone on the floor and the caller saying "Chester, go get Janet".

This idea of leveraging upon an animal's natural predisposition makes a lot of sense. We reasoned that because horses have evolved as prey animals they are super-sensitive to potential danger which would be a desirable trait for a guide animal.

Continuing our research we discovered the differences between Service Animals and Therapy animals, the controversy surrounding emotional support animals and the types of animals appropriate for flying in USA commercial aircraft. Here is a summary of what we learned.

Functions of Service Animals

Reading the text of the Americans with Disabilities Act (ADA) teaches some interesting facts. To get the full rights of public access, the handler must have a diagnosable disability and the Service animal must perform a specific, measurable service. There are many types of Service Animals:

- **Guide Animals** – Dogs (and now horses) have been successfully used as guides for the blind.

- **Mobility Aid Animals** – Horses and dogs are used to pull wheelchairs for people who cannot walk unaided due to Multiple Sclerosis, Paralysis, broken limbs, or morbid obesity. Mobility Animals are also used to retrieve objects and steady people with balance-related disabilities such as inner-ear disorders and Cerebral Palsy and Multiple Sclerosis.

- **Medical Alert Animals** – Does, horses, pigs and cats are currently used to provide alerts for the impending onset of life-threatening medical conditions such as epilepsy, insulin shock, stroke and various neurological seizures.

- **Signal Animals** - Dogs cats, monkeys and pigs are currently recognized as performing legitimate services for the hearing impaired. These services include warning about noise-related danger signals (i.e. sirens, car horns) and also include alerting to everyday signals such as telephone calls and doorbells.

- **Tranquility Animals** – A Tranquility Animal performs the service of moderating or maintaining bodily functions such as heart rate and blood pressure, and clinical studies confirm that Tranquility Animals provide a measurable service to the elderly, and those with severe emotional disorders. The only training required for most Tranquility Animals is basic housebreaking and obedience, and their presence alone is sufficient to perform the service to their handler. I was surprised to find that a Tranquility Animal can cross-over from Therapy Animal to Service Animal (gaining access rights under the ADA) if their presence causes a consistent, measurable change in the physiological status of their handler.

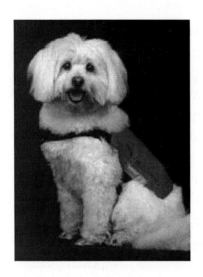

A Hearing assistance dog

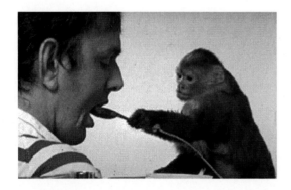

A Mobility Aid monkey

Helping Hands
Monkey Helpers for the Disabled has grown from an

innovative idea to a thriving non-profit organization that offers independence and hope to individuals with severe disabilities across the country. Helping Hands: Monkey Helpers for the Disabled trained and placed the first monkey as helper and a companion to a paralyzed individual in 1979. From the beginning, Helping Hands mission has been to provide assistance to people with the greatest need: people who have become quadriplegic (paralyzed from the neck down) as a result of an accident, injury, or disease. There are currently over 200,000 people in the United States who have become paralyzed as a result of a spinal cord injury, with an additional 12,000–15,000 new injuries occurring each year. Most people are between the ages of 16-26 at the time of their injury. Helping Hands' programs have been developed to raise and train capuchin monkeys to be assistive and treasured live-in companions, and to provide support to monkey helpers and their severely handicapped human partners throughout their lives together.

Helping Hands monkeys transform the lives of their quadriplegic companions. Small miracles happen every day. There are the miracles of hugs, of a helping hand, of love and companionship. Year after year, the monkeys are the miracles that empower the lives of disabled individuals.

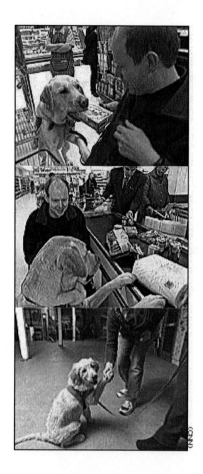

A mobility aid dog on-duty

Surprisingly there is no governing body for training and certifying service animals and the ADA guarantees the rights of any disabled person to train their own Service Animal. Owner-trained Service Animals have equal rights to those that are trained by volunteer or charitable organizations and the ADA supersedes State laws, such as the California law requiring licensing for guide dog trainers.

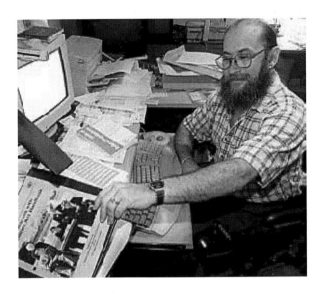

Fred Shotz, an ADA advocate uses self-trained Service Dogs

Dr. Fred Shotz, an advocate for disabled rights, trains his dogs to pull his wheelchair, chariot style.

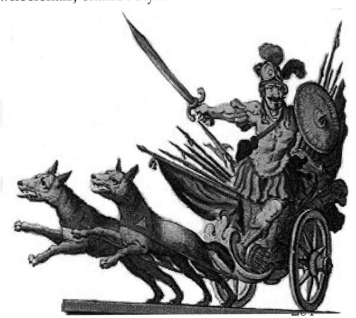

Rights of Service Animal Users

Knowing that the ADA guarantees the access right of a Service Animal to any public place, we were not aware that the law does not require any type of certification for a Service Animal and that nobody is entitled to impose any standards of performance for a Service Animal.

I learned that it is the handler, not the Service Animal, who has the Civil Rights, and that it is a criminal act to interfere with the access rights of a Service Animal. This interference includes asking for any type of certification, asking the disabled person to prove that their animal performs a service, or publishing false or misleading information about Service Animals.

When we first began training with Karen Clark, she told us many stories about being challenged when using her guide dog. Confident in her access rights, Karen responds to the challenge
"You can't bring an animal in here!" with the calm reply of *"Yes, I can"*, as she continues to go about her business.

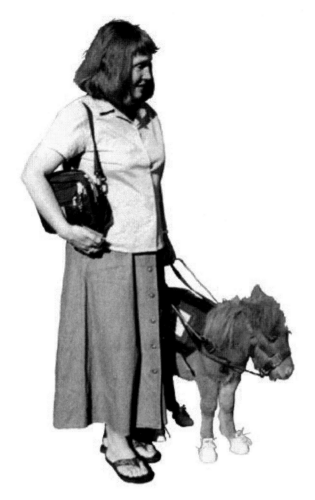

Karen Clark with Cuddles

Sadly, we learned that all Service Animal users must constantly protect their rights against challenges by those who don't know the law. There are organizations that sells T-shirts to remind the public, and many of the shirts make it very clear that many Service Animal users have problems with public ignorance of their access rights.

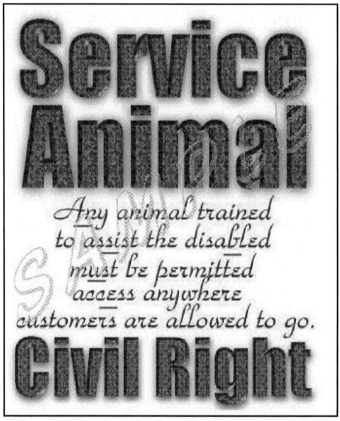

T-shirt reminding the public about Civil Rights Violations

It was especially surprising that discrimination still exists in view of the penalties. The ADA was written to vigorously protect the Civil Rights of Service Animal handlers and the Department of Justice provides for a $50,000 fine for the first offense to anyone who interferes with a Service Animal handler's right to public access.

Civil court awards commonly run high when outraged juries award punitive damages against those who conspire to deprive an individual (or any group of Service Animal users) of their Civil Rights. In Raleigh, North Carolina, a restaurant owner who denied access to a Guide Animal was sued for Civil Rights violations. The outraged public boycotted the restaurant, eventually forcing it to go out of business.

In sum, the ADA was created to protect disabled people from constant challenges and harassment in their daily life.

Next, let's take a look at the different species that are used as Service Animals. We will then contrast a Service Animals with a Therapy animal and attempt to clarify the differences in services and access rights.

Types of Service Animals

Service Animals may be of any species, so long as the animal can be shown to perform a measurable service to a disabled person.

Service Dogs – Dogs are very versatile and are used as guides, alert animals, mobility animals and therapeutic animals.

Service pigs – Small Pot-bellied pigs are recognized to perform the services of an Alert Animal, and they are a preferred choice for disabled people who are allergic to dogs.

Service monkeys – Monkeys are very valuable assets to this with paralyzed limbs and monkeys are trained to provide a variety of complex services such as depositing fees into bus fare receptacles.

Service cats – Cats are used as alert animals, assisting deaf people.

Service horses –. A Service Horse may be used to provide stability and to pull a wheelchair.

Service Birds – Birds have been shown to perform services to the disabled, primarily by serving as Alert Animals for the hearing   impaired.

Therapy Animals

While a Service Animal must perform a measurable service to the disabled, a Therapy Animal does not have to perform any identifiable service. Therapy animals are often used for individuals who have serious mental disabilities such as fear of flying or emotional trauma resulting from a mugging. For this class of the disabled, the Therapy Animals need only provide the person with a "sense of comfort", which is not a measurable service as defined by the ADA.

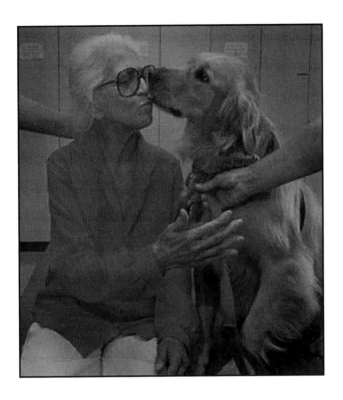

Therapy Dog on-duty

The use of Therapy animals generally requires an approved American Psychological Association (APA) diagnosis from a qualified Mental health professional (Psychologist or Psychiatrist). These diagnoses may include:

Phobias – Those with fear of open places (Agoraphobia), emotionally traumatized crime victims and those with a fear of flying may use an Emotional Support Animal. For example, a crime victim with a fear of being attacked might have a large therapy dog to make them feel safe in public. **Neurological Disorders** –Sometimes therapy animals are used to assist with the care of People with Autism.

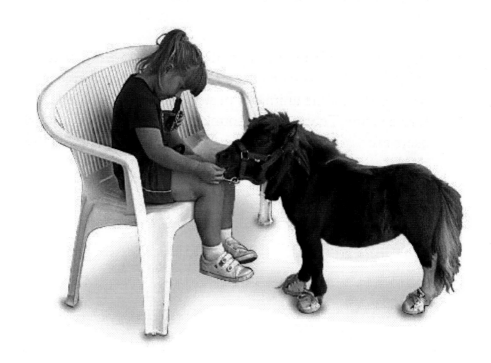

A companion pony for a child

The Therapy Animal may not be protected under the Americans with Disabilities Act, because it cannot be shown to provide a measurable service. Rather, the benefits of Therapy Animals are the subjective reports of diagnosed anxiety, which may not be quantifiably measurable.

Any Therapy Animal that cannot be shown to perform a measurable service does not have the same guaranteed rights to public access as a Service Animal. However, one important exception to this rule are Tranquility and Emotional Support Animals whose owners can demonstrate a consistent, measurable physiological response to the use of the animal.

For example, if the presence of an Emotional Support animal can be shown to decrease heart rate or blood pressure, then the animal is performing the legitimate services of a Therapeutic Animal and Therapeutic Animal users are protected under the ADA and afforded all rights to public access.

Horse Selection

 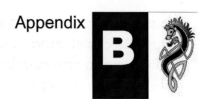
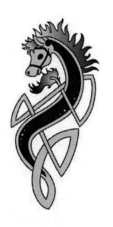

Field intelligence testing for Guide Horse Candidates

Intelligence in horses is quite different from other domestic animals. Because horses have evolved as prey animals, the intelligence of a horse is quite different from that of a predatory animal, and different metrics must be used as a measure. We generally look to quantify equine intelligence along three dimensions:

Scope of learning – Determining the cognitive ability of a horse to solve increasingly complex problems.

Rate of learning - A quantitative measure of the time required for the horse to learn the task.

Retention of learning – The ability of the horse to remember the learned behavior.

The intelligence of horses is often represented as an evenly distributed bell curve, with approximately 80% of horses falling within two standard deviations from the mean. This distribution of equine intelligence suggests that it is possible to develop a field test to identify those horses with superior intelligence. While it is not practical to administer clinical testing in the field, we developed a reliable field test for measuring equine intelligence.

To be accurate, a field test of intelligence must measure the alertness of the horse and manner in which the horse interacts with the environment. The field test consists of the following areas:

Ear reflex index – Alert horses with a high degree of ear motility tend to be more intelligent and a measure of the ear reflex index can discern the intelligence of the horse.
Pressure Response - Measuring sensitivity and response to pressure can often reveal the hoses intelligence. Intelligent horses respond quickly and decisively to applied pressure.
Response to socialization – Intelligent horses have mastered equine social behavior and display the proper "etiquette" when interacting with other horses and people.
Umveg testing – Intelligent horses are able to navigate a detour to achieve a goal.

While these tests are somewhat subjective and difficult to quantify, they provide a fairly accurate measurement of equine intelligence. To show how each metric is gathered, let's examine the details of each field test.

Ear motion Index

The first phase of the field intelligence test measures the relative ear motion of the horse. All horses have a range of motion of 170 degrees, and intelligent horses demonstrate frequent and independent ear motion. In the field, two trainers administer the ear motion test.

One stands near the left front of the horse and the other person orients themselves at the right rear. As the trainers walk around the horse, the intelligent horse will follow the people with their ears, tracking their motion independently from the other ear. A less alert horse will remain with their ears in the "neutral position, with the ears facing 30 degrees forward, while the intelligent horse will demonstrate rapid and independent ear motion.

Pressure Response

Many horse trainers rely on the "release of pressure" method to train a horse. In nature, horses are programmed to move into pressure as a survival technique. For example, if a wolf clamped-down on the horse's nose, the horse will not pull away and risk having its nose torn. Rather, the horse will move "into" the pressure, thereby decreasing the chance of loosing the appendage.

Horse trainers have long known that the mark of a smart horse is their responsiveness to pressure as evidenced by their direct and purposeful moving "into" physical pressure. To test this in the field, the trainer will spread their fingers and press hard on the side of the horse, directly below the withers. An intelligent horse will immediately lean-into the trainers hand, while the less intelligent horse will either fail to respond to the pressure or move away from the source of the pressure. The exception to this rule would be a horse that has already been trained to move away from pressure. We were testing horses that had not been exposed to any training or attempts at behavior modification.

Response to Socialization

As a herd animal, horses communicate frequently with other horses and learn a variety of social interaction skills. Their mastery of social etiquette can be measured, and the more intelligent horse learns quickly to response to social cues in an appropriate manner. The simplest test of horse socialization skill is the process of greeting. To illustrate, let's review how two horses meet.

Two horses always approach each other with their necks extended and their head's bowed. They then touch noses and exchange scents by blowing short blasts of air into each other's nostrils. This blowing of air is done is short puffs, about two per second until the scent is acknowledged.

This greeting is the human equivalent of exchanging business cards, and is analogous to dogs introducing each other by sniffing the tail area.

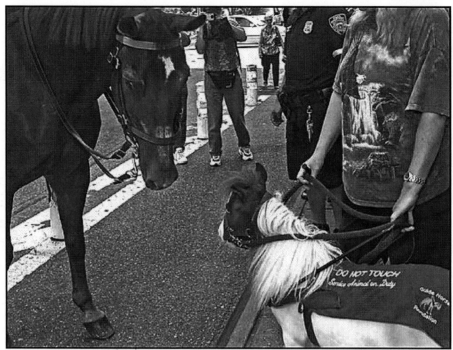

Once the introduction is completed, the horses move to the next phase, where they "squeal" at each other. Horses are very concerned about their status in the horse hierarchy, and in this phase the horses will challenge each other, sometimes striking out with their front legs. This behavior will continue until one of the horses will show signs of submission.

In the field, the trainer can gauge the horse's mastery of social etiquette by greeting the horse as a fellow equine. The trainer approaches the horse from the front, places their face adjacent to the horse's snout and blows short puff of air up the horse's nostrils. An intelligent horse will always display a visible reaction at this greeting and will widen their eyes and point both of their each straight forward. A less intelligent horse will not respond with the appropriate actions.

Umveg Testing

Umveg is the process of taking a detour in order to reach a goal. In horses, the ability to do an umveg is an undisputed sign of superior intelligence. For a field test, the horse is lead to one side of an open-ended ten foot wire fence and given a treat. Next, the horse is lead around to the other side of the fence and a treat is place into a bowl directly opposite the horse. An intelligent horse will turn away from the food and circumnavigate the fence to get the food, while a less intelligent horse will stand on the opposite side of the fence and paw the ground. In practice, the more intelligent the horse, the faster they will recognize the need to move away from the treat to get around the fence.

Using these testing principles we were able to judge the horse's suitability to enter the training program. There were other factors to consider also as the horse must also be serviceably sound and healthy. We relied on our veterinarian's judgment as to the horse's physical suitability for a life as a service animal.

Owning a Miniature Horse

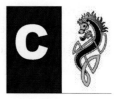

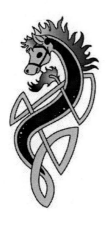

Everyone agrees that miniature horses are cute and friendly, causing hundreds of requests each month from people who want to have one as a pet. Before considering buying or adopting a miniature horse, make sure that you are in a position to make a lifelong commitment to provide a safe and healthy home for a horse. Miniature horses are real horses and they have many of the same care requirements as full size horses.

Are You Ready to be Horse Poor?

Responsible horse owners understand that it can take significant funds to properly care for a miniature horse. While the term "Horse Poor" was originally coined to refer to large horse ownership, the same concept can apply to miniature horse owners. Individuals that spend all their disposable income on

216

their horses are commonly referred to as "Horse Poor". Once you make the decision to have a horse you have to be prepared to provide for its daily needs.

Sadly, because pet quality miniature horses are inexpensive they are often purchased by individuals who don't realize that the purchase price is like a down payment on a horse. It's a tiny fraction of the cost of keeping and caring for the horse for its natural lifespan. When a new horse owner doesn't have the financial resources to properly care for a miniature horse, everyone suffers, especially the little horses.

Remember, owning a miniature horse is a huge responsibility because of their longevity. It is not uncommon for a properly maintained miniature horse to live to be 35, and in some unusual cases, more than 40 years old. Unless you are prepared to make a long term commitment to a miniature horse, miniature horse ownership may not be right for you.

Is Your Home Suitable for a Miniature Horse?

Before buying a miniature horse, you should verify that you meet the minimum requirements:

- **Grazing Space** – Horses need room to run and graze. Miniature horses don't live indoors so they need a suitable outside living space. A half acre of pasture is the minimum space required to keep a miniature horse happy and stress free.

- **Horse Care Experience** – If you don't have previous experience caring for and handling horses it would be wise to take the time to learn as much as possible before you bring home a miniature equine. Reading books on horse care and horse behavior is an excellent start. You would also benefit from taking the time to visit horse farms and participating in hands-on lessons grooming and handling horses. Establishing a relationship with a local instructor will give you someone you trust to call for advice when there are problems with your new horses.

- **Zoning** - The neighborhood must be zoned for livestock or exotic animals. Miniature horses are considered livestock so they can not be maintained in areas zoned against livestock. Occasionally neighborhoods that permit exotic animals will accept miniature horses as exotic pets. People often try to keep horses in areas without proper zoning only to learn that they have to remove them to comply with the zoning regulations.

- **Friends** - Horses are herd animals that get lonely without at least one miniature horse companion. To be kind to your miniature horse you should always have at least two miniature horses. A horse kept alone will always long for equine companionship, sometimes going so far as to escape to go in search of other horses.

- **Funds** – While routine Veterinary care for a miniature horse is similar in cost to that required for a dog or cat, all pets can be expensive if they need more than routine Veterinary care. Life saving Veterinary treatment and surgery can cost many thousands of dollars. Preparation for a possible crisis can help prevent the heartache of not

218

being able to give your horse the care it needs to survive a life threatening illness or injury.

Once you are certain that you can provide the proper care and a suitable home for a miniature horse it's time to find a horse or two.

Finding a Miniature Horse Pet

Miniature horses are not rare so it is not necessary to spend thousands of dollars to buy a show quality miniature horse if you only want a pet or companion. Here are some suggested venues where you can find miniature horses for sale:

- **Regular Horse Auctions** - You can often buy a nice miniature horse at regular horse auctions and get the added benefit of saving a life. Many of the horses sold at auctions go to slaughter.

- **Miniature Horse Auctions** – There are miniature horse auctions all over the country where a healthy registered miniature horse can often be purchased for less than $350.

- **Horse Rescue Organizations** - Every year thousands of unwanted miniature horses and ponies are slaughtered, and you can help by adopting a neglected or abused miniature horse. Many unwanted miniature horses are saved by charitable equine rescue organizations and are available to be adopted for a nominal fee.

- **Miniature Horse Breeders** – There are hundreds of farms that breed and sell miniature horses to the public. A local breeder can often be a valuable source of information and help with the care of your new miniature horse. An Internet search can provide you with contact info for a breeder in your area.

Miniature Horse Prices

Rising from obscurity, miniature horses have enjoyed large swings in popularity over the past 50 years. From the initial interest in 1962 when tiny ponies grazed on the White House lawn to sad periods where over abundant ponies were sent to the killers for meat.

Because miniature horses are hardy and require little pasture, breeders with significant acreage were able to run herds of hundreds of tiny horses, flooding the market with thousands of miniature horses driving the prices down.

There is a wide variety in miniature horse prices ranging from over $100,000 to less than $5. In Great Britain, the Dartmoor National Park is known for its hundreds of square miles full of free range ponies that can be purchased for less than the cost of a taxi ride.

Each year the ponies are swept from the moors and brought to an auction sale. Because of the high-costs of equine ownership in the UK, prices fell at one point to below $3.00 US per pony. Today, the killers buy most of the Dartmoor ponies for the dinner tables of Europe.

However, there is that rare, perfect miniature horse that will sell for a large sum of money. Producing a perfect specimen often requires breeding hundreds of mares and the successful breeder is rewarded with huge rewards. Among the top-selling miniature horses we have seen:

- **Lazy N's Boogerman** – This tiny stallion sold for $110,000 at the NFC farm dispersal sale in the 1980s.

- **Boones Little Buckaroo** – This little horse was reported to have sold for $100,000 in 1983.

Celebrity purchases also drive up prices as was the case when Michael Jackson and Cher purchased miniature horses for their estates.

Ironically, every year hundreds of unwanted horses are euthanized or slaughtered for food while the top champions continue to command huge sums from wealthy horse owners.

Today a buyer can purchase a pet-quality miniature horse for under $200 or spend over $100,000 for a national champion. However, when purchasing a miniature horse you might want to ensure that your money does not go to breeders who do not ensure good homes for all their baby ponies.

In summary, pet quality miniature horses are abundant and it is not necessary to spend thousands of dollars on a show-quality miniature horse if you are not interested in showing. We highly recommend that you spend your money to save a discarded or abused miniature horse. You will have a noble friend for many decades.

Consider Adopting a Dartmoor Pony

The Dartmoor National Park in southwestern England is home to thousands of semi-wild miniature ponies. Over a million yearly visitors flock to the moors to see the wild herds of wonderful miniature horses running free in one of the most scenic areas of England. At roadside stops, the semi-domesticated ponies will come up, begging for snacks.

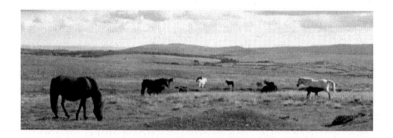

The wild Dartmoor ponies

Dartmoor ponies range in size from riding sized to those under 28 inches tall. Many resemble the American miniature horses, with the notable exception that none have the dwarf characteristics associated with some miniature horse breeding programs.

The Dartmoor Pony Society notes that the Dartmoor ponies have been present on the moors for nearly one thousand years:

"Though there have been few references through the centuries to the ponies in old writings the earliest is said to have been in about the 11th century."

According to other scholars, the earliest reference to the Dartmoor Pony appeared in 1012 in the Will of a Saxon Bishop, Aelfwold of Crediton.

The Dartmoor Pony is an official miniaturized horse breed and registered in the UK Rare Breed Trust. There are several breed societies and registries associated with Dartmoor ponies.

- Dartmoor Pony - (As listed in the UK Rare Breeds Survival Trust)

- The Dartmoor Pony Registry of America

- Dartmoor Pony Society

Don and I have visited Dartmoor several times and the unbelievable beauty of the free ponies is undermined by the fact that many of these sweet ponies will wind up being slaughtered within a year.

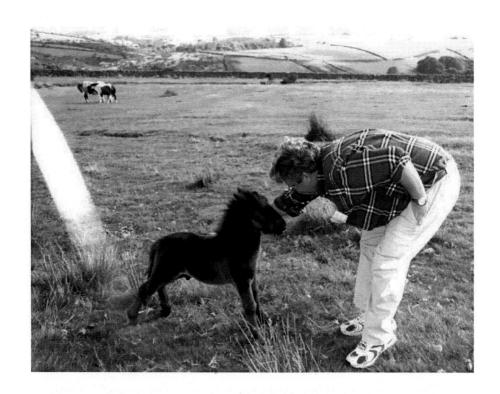

Tiny ponies can be purchased in Dartmoor for only a few dollars

Many of the smaller miniature ponies at Dartmoor are well within the height requirements of the USA Miniature Horse Registries, yet the British miniature pony breeders report that dwarfism, dystocia and abortions are as low as that with large breed horses. They are very friendly, even in their wild state.

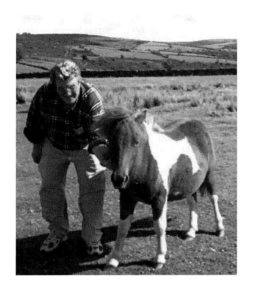

Tiny ponies roam free across hundreds of square miles

Each year the ponies are swept from the moors and brought to an auction sale. Because of the high-costs of equine ownership in the UK, prices fell at one point to below $3.00 US dollars per pony. Today, the killers buy most of the Dartmoor ponies for the dinner tables of France.

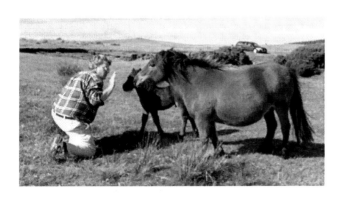

We highly recommend that anyone consider traveling to England take the time to adopt a wonderful Dartmoor pony. The shipping may cost hundreds of dollars, but you get a wonderful vacation and the chance to save the life of an innocent pony.

The Sad Sweeping of the Moor

Every year, weanlings are swept from the Moor and auctioned. According to the official Dartmoor National Park web site, many of the ponies produced were unwanted and sold to the dining pleasure of French dinner tables:

"Many people will be familiar with the sad images of unwanted and unsaleable Dartmoor ponies in the last few years being offered at pony auctions around the moor and often selling for just a few £'s if they could find a buyer at all. Nobody wanted them, they were unhandled and taken straight from their mothers and considered of no worth."

According to an article by the BBC, the miniature horses face a grim fate each fall, many going into recipes:

"A drop in demand for the ponies from riders and meat traders has seen prices fall from £40 several years ago to as low as £2." "One farmer, Neil Cole, said: "People with a lot of ponies are just shooting them or giving them the big hit. There's literally nothing else we can do with the Dartmoor ponies."

Miniature Horse Owner Medical Responsibility

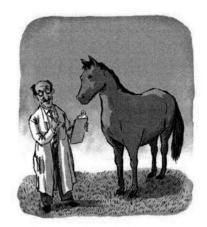

With 21st Century technology it is possible to save a sick or injured miniature horse what would otherwise have to be euthanized.

Examples include:

- **Broken Legs** - For example, today's technology allows miniature horses to survive broken legs. Later we will tell you the story of the successful treatment of a miniature horse with a broken leg, but note that the surgery may cost as much as $8,000.

- **Colic** - Surgical techniques can now save horses from serious gastric impactions.

- **Foaling Surgery** - The regular use of foaling hospitals can save the lives of mare and foals. This includes Ceasarian sections for foal delivery and medical techniques to save premature miniature horse foals.

- **Geriatric Care** - Advancements in Veterinary technology now allow many of the same treatments used for elderly humans including arthritis medications and special foods for elderly horses whose teeth have worn out.

Even though miniature horses are cheaper than most large dogs to feed, vaccinate and maintain, responsible miniature horse owners will keep a reserve fund of at least $5,000 to ensure life-saving surgery for acute illness and injury. Sometimes an innocent pony is killed because the owner cannot afford proper medical treatment. It's not unusual to hear owners lament,

"Surgery is out of the question because of the cost. It is about $5000. As much as it breaks our hearts, we just can't afford that."

Over the past 50 years, midget pony breeders deliberately introduced deadly genetic anomalies into their bloodlines, making breeding a miniature horse in the USA a risky proposition.

Now that we have a good background in miniature horse ownership, let's look at some structures that you can build to keep your ponies safe from harsh elements.

Miniature barns for Miniature Horses

While you can keep miniature horses in a full size stable it's not necessary. Especially if space is limited a miniature size barn will serve the purpose without using up precious grazing areas.

We designed several miniature horse barn shelters for the specific needs of miniature horses. They adequately provide a complete shelter for the horses and are attractive additions to the horse's living area.

Victorian Style Miniature Horse Barn

This is a practical miniature horse barn, combining the Victorian style with the utility of a well-vented roof. This miniature horse barn design retains heat and provides shade, all while allowing for the proper ventilation that is critical to the health of the Miniature Horse.

Dimensions:	8 feet wide by 8 feet long
	3.5 feet to gables and 5 feet at apex of roof
Materials Cost:	Approximately $240
Construction Time:	Approximately 45 hours

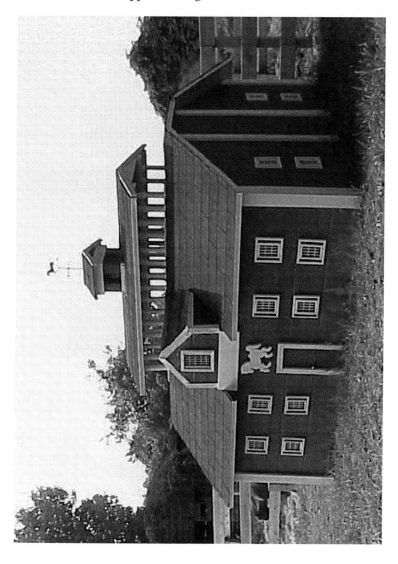

Carolina Model Miniature Horse Barn

This pragmatic miniature horse barn combines elegant style with easy access. The slanted roof design provides adequate ventilation while providing easy access for both the miniature horse and the groom. The custom-designed upper hinged door allows a six-foot human access to the barn for cleaning while providing warmth in the winter and shade in the summer months. This miniature horse barn design includes the ideal combination of easy construction and safe miniature horse barn design.

Specifications:

Dimensions:	*8 feet wide by 8 feet long*
	Four feet to gables and 6.5 feet at apex of roof
Materials Cost:	*Approximately $190*
Construction time:	*Approximately 25 hours*

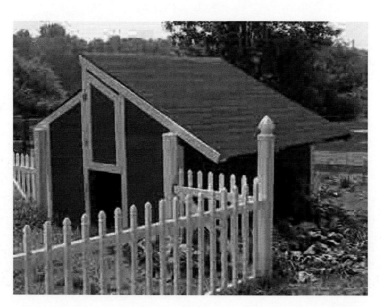

Herd Style Miniature Horse Barn

This miniature horse barn is designed for protection from the elements. The design is ideal for protecting miniature horses of a variety of heights providing warmth in the winter and protection from thunderstorms.

Specifications:

Dimensions:	*8 feet wide by 12 feet long*
	Four feet to 2nd tier and 6.5 feet at apex of roof
Materials Cost:	*Approximately $290*
Construction time:	*Approximately 45 hours*

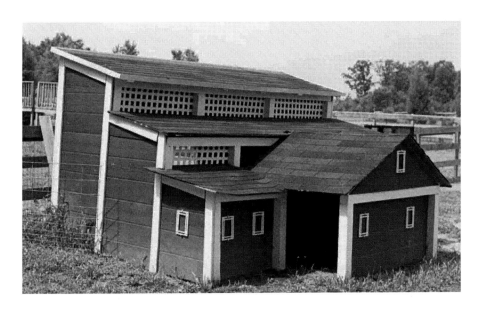

Unfortunately, not all breeders take all of the necessary precautions to minimize the risk to the miniature mare and foal. The losses of some miniature horse breeders are shocking, some ranging as high as one-third of their entire breeding population.

It all boils down to proper evaluation of the breeders and the individual that you are interested in buying. Try to support breeders who keep the best interest of their animals as a priority!

Finding a Breeder

Not all miniature horse breeders are alike, with wide variations in concern for pre-natal care and careful animal husbandry.

Some of the most reckless miniature horse breeders deliberately breed dwarf miniature horses without any regard for the extreme suffering of these sad genetic mutations. Others ignore the high risk of miniature horse birthing problems and fail to use proper precautions sometimes leading to the unnecessary suffering and death of mares and foals. For more details, see the Appendix on Miniature horse breeding.

You may want to buy your miniature horse from a quality miniature horse breeder who carefully researches their pedigrees, out-crosses their bloodlines and makes proper investment in medical care for foaling mares.

You also may want to ensure that you do not buy a miniature horse with dwarf ancestors. Many of the horses offered for sale may carry genetic markers for dwarfism. Even if you not planning on breeding your miniature horse, you may not want to subsidize an irresponsible breeder, there by contributing to the

232

suffering of dead broodmares and the dwarf horse by-products that might be produced by breeding stock with dwarf ancestors.

Avoiding Dwarf Producers

While many believe that it is impossible to breed miniature horses without producing an occasional dwarf, you should avoid sellers who deliberately breed dwarves and those who do not invest in out-crossing bloodlines.

Dwarfism is rare in the large horse breeds, but quite common in miniature horses, especially among reckless breeders. A dwarf horse often leads a short and painful life, yet there are some miniature horse breeders who continue to produce dwarf horses in large numbers. These miniature horse breeders will go to great lengths to hide a dwarf horse from public viewing, yet many continue to place profit above suffering, and continue to use dwarf horses as breeding stock.

As mentioned earlier some people note that miniature horses in North America have been deliberately contaminated with dwarfism genes and the astronomical rates of foal death and birth defects are far less in foreign programs that never deliberately bred exclusively for small size with unhealthy dwarves.

Miniature horse buyers who do not want their purchase to contribute to the death of other miniatures horses won't consider buying a miniature horse from breeders who deliberately breed dwarves or breed miniature horses with dwarf ancestors. There appears to be evidence that historical breeders have deliberately introduced dwarfism into some USA miniature horses.

While there is a great debate about the cause and prevention of miniature horse dwarfism, many doctors cite a clear link to genetics and the frequency of dwarf horse production.

The suffering of these tiny dwarf horses is shocking. Many live for only a few days, while others may suffer for many years with crippling leg deformities and other serious health problems.

Miniature Horse Spaying and Gelding

Some experts believe that only professional breeders should keep stallions and fertile mares. Here are the main issues surrounding miniature horse fertility and behavior.

Gelding

All stallions can be aggressive, and the miniature horse is no exception. With the glut of miniature horses in the USA, most miniature horse owners choose to geld their colts as soon as they are mature enough. Stallions will fight with other stallions, become aggressive with handlers and mares and cause danger for small children. The gelding procedure can be performed by a veterinarian for a nominal fee, and this simple operation will resolve a number of behavioral issues including:

- **Aggression** - Stallions are naturally territorial and aggressive and may bite and kick without warning.

- **Manners** - Geldings are not hormone driven and can peacefully co-exist with mares and do not require segregation like a stallion does.

Spaying

With the glut of miniature horses on the market, many miniature horse owners are choosing to spay their mares, for many reasons. Even when segregated from stallions, a mare's estrus cycles can cause unpredictable behavior. And it only takes one breach in the fence for stallions and mares to intermingle. We have been advised that in some areas spaying can now be done via arthroscopic surgery (laparoscopic surgery) at less expense than ever before.

Spaying the Dwarf Miniature Horse

Spaying is a common practice for dwarf miniature mares. Spaying a mare with dwarf characteristics will guarantee that the dwarf characteristics won't be carried forward to another generation.

Equine Dwarfism

 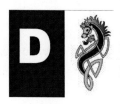

According to the American Miniature Horse Association (One of the more popular registries in the USA) small size is important:

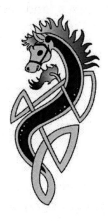

"The ideal Miniature Horse of today, according to the American Miniature Horse Association's Standard of Perfection, must be small (standing at or less than 34 inches tall as measured from the last hairs of the mane,)"

Because the smaller ponies brought higher prices, some breeders became obsessed with reducing the size of their product, many bred exclusively for size, ignoring the genetic anomalies that accompany breeding exclusively for size.

Some famous stud horses such as Bond Tiny Tim (only 19" tall) were believed to be dwarf horses with leg deformities, but were still bred passing on potentially crippling genetic mutations.

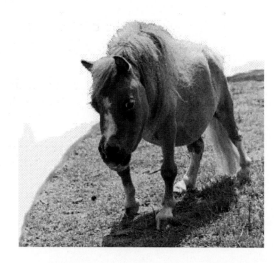

Severe dwarf miniature horses may live for only a few days, while others may suffer for many years with crippling leg deformities and other serious health problems. Fortunately, some caring people will adopt and attempt to rehabilitate a crippled dwarf horse.

If you do a Google search on "dwarf horse memorial" you can see photos of severely deformed miniature horses and read tributes from their heartbroken owners.

Bluebell

"I've got the perfect horse for you", the caller explained. *"She is only 21 inches tall, very smart, and I'd like you to have her. She has a few problems with her hooves but you can get them straightened-out very easily."*

I thanked the woman for her generosity and arranged for "Bluebell" to be transported to the Guide Horse Foundation. When she arrived, I was shocked. Bluebell was an adorable blue-gray filly with bright blue eyes and a friendly personality, but I had never seen a horse with such horrible conformation.

Her back was roached, I could count her ribs at 30 paces and her backbone protruded more than an inch.

Her bite was way off and her vocal cords were misplaced, such that she can never knicker or whinny. But the real horror was her deformed legs.

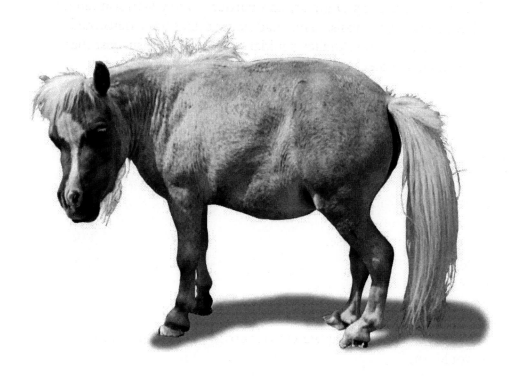

Bluebell hooves could have been more properly described as "horns". They were over 6 inches long and curved under her body like giant Elf shoes. She could still run but it was clear that she had some serious health issues and would never become a Guide Horse.

Our Vet, Dr. Chris O'Malley and Farrier, Danny Harmon did not have a good prognosis. They had never seen such a deformed horse before. Dr. O'Malley's initial reaction was to suggest that we euthanize the feeble little pony.

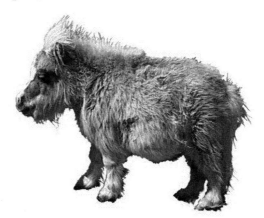

Having been taught to take people at face value, I was known for trusting a person until proven otherwise. Now I was cursing my gullibility.

The woman knew that we would provide the health care that she would not.

Of course, I could not allow Bluebell to be killed. Danny and Chris gave the prognosis.

"If I work with Chris we can tear-down the horns and attempt to rebuild a set of new feet. He will need special trimming and custom hoof attachments every week for at least four years, and possibly for life. The total cost will be about $1,500 per year, and I can't guarantee that she will ever walk normally. To start, we're going to cast her legs down to her hooves and make the cast into splints because her joints are so weak," Danny explained.

Because of this huge expense, Bluebell was withdrawn from the Guide Horse list and became a rescue project.

Bluebell was a very smart and personable pony and took the painful treatments without complaint. She was placed on painkillers and arthritis medicine, but it made me cry every time her feet were adjusted.

She would lie down bravely for the new hoof attachments and then hobble in great pain, taking tiny tentative steps until she grew comfortable with her new attachments.

Because of her off-bite she could not eat grass normally and Dr. O'Malley recommended a special feed to allow her to gain weight.

Every two weeks I watched Bluebell suffer as she adjusted to her treatments and my empathy began to turn to anger. I was angry that Bluebell hooves had been neglected for such a long time, and outraged that people might breed these ponies into a life of suffering.

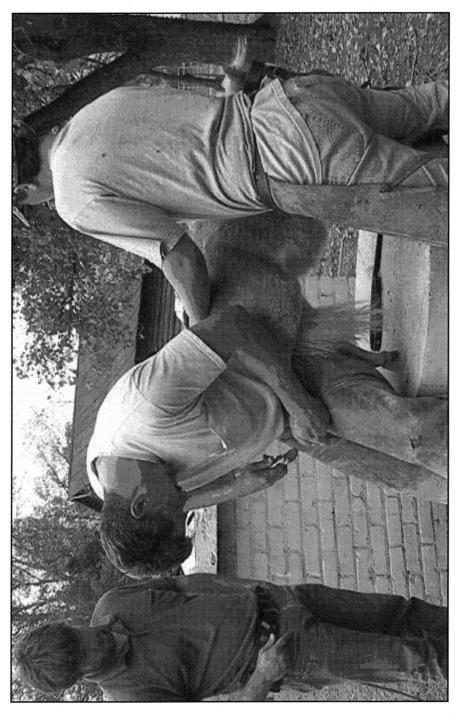

241

As the years passed we were able to control Bluebell's pain and gradually straighten her front legs. Bluebell was examined by four orthopedic surgeons who said that corrective surgery was not an option, and that her deformed spine made it impossible for Dr. O'Malley to straighten her back legs.

Gradually Bluebell became the head mare of our dwarf colony and during her pain-free times she started to act like a normal horse. It was both heartwarming and hilarious to see Bluebell flirting with the stallions, and occasionally bucking and playing with her friends.

Sometimes when Danny came by for a treatment he wondered-aloud why we spent so much money on her. Don was concerned that he might give up and offered Danny a $100 bill for the first time Bluebell cantered. Don thought it was a safe bet because she spent much of her day lying down, grazing on her side, and only moving a few feet at a time. One day in 2004, we were all gathering for Bluebell's scheduled treatment when we witnessed a remarkable event. Almost as if on-cue, Bluebell galloped across her pasture! Don, always true to his word, began peeling twenty dollar bills from his wallet!

Today Bluebell is a relatively comfortable 5 year-old. She will never run and play with the other ponies, but she loves her dwarf chow and enjoys being groomed and spoiled with attention. For now she is leading a quality life, but someday the arthritis and deformities will cause her unimaginable pain and we will be forced to have Bluebell euthanized.

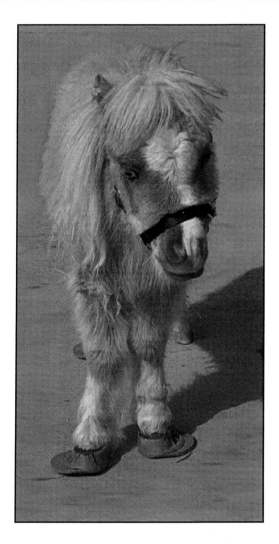

Bluebell is a special dwarf because of her wonderful nature. She recently adopted a dwarf foal named BeeBee and they have become inseparable. Bluebell and BeeBee are always side-by-side and most amazingly, Bluebell developed milk for her new baby!

BeeBee was adopted by the Guide Horse Foundation because he had contracted strangles and his owner could not afford to save his life. BeeBee spent several weeks in the horse hospital, receiving a tracheotomy and getting treatment for the huge blisters caused by this potentially fatal horse disease.

Upon his return from the hospital, BeeBee was weaned from his mother and he joined the dwarf herd.

It is not unknown for horses who adopt babies to produce milk for them, and this serves to demonstrate Bluebell's huge affection for her tiny friend.

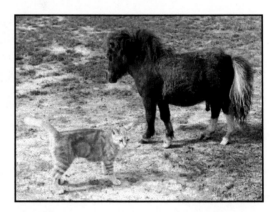

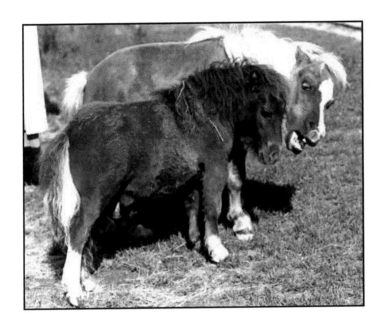

BeeBee and Bluebell

Popular
Horse Sayings

 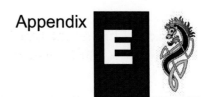

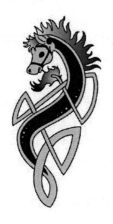

Horse reference phrases are commonly used in daily conversation. Here are some of our favorites.

Have you heard these phrases before?

He looks like he's been rode hard and put up wet - Referring to a horse that has foundered by not being properly cooled-off after riding, a lame person.

Nobody will ever notice it on a galloping horse - Don't be too self-conscious about your appearance.

If wishes were horses, beggars would ride - Poor folks dream, rich folks do.

He would steal the bridle off a nightmare. He will steal anything that he can get his hands on.

She could eat an apple through a picket fence. Small enough to reach her muzzle through a picket fence.

Don't look a gift horse in the mouth. Don't be ungrateful.

Straight from the horse's mouth. Information that comes from the top.

Long in the tooth. Calling someone old because old horses have long teeth.

Winning by a nose. Refers to a close horse race.

Down the homestretch. Nearing the finish as in a horse race.

For want of a nail a shoe was lost, for want of a shoe a horse was lost, for want of a horse a rider was lost, for want of a rider a army was lost, for want of an army a battle was lost, for want of a battle the war was lost, for want of the war the kingdom was lost, and all for the want of a little horseshoe nail.
--Benjamin Franklin

About Janet Burleson

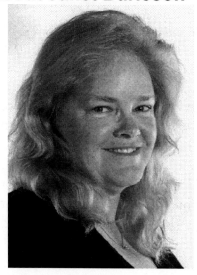 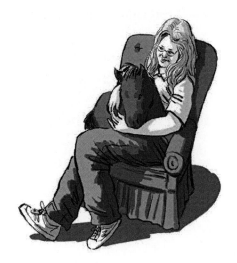

As a lifelong horse training enthusiast, Janet Burleson has experimented with hundreds of horse behavior challenges. With four decades of horse teaching experience, she is the pioneering horse trainer that developed the Guide horse training program.

Janet is also one of the world's pioneering horse trainers, having developed the successful Guide Horse Foundation donating her time and effort to train miniature horses to guide the blind. **www.guidehorse.com**

As an expert Web design consultant Janet provides high level web consulting services that improve the market status of Fortune 500 companies including web search rank positioning, keyword optimization, web content optimization, web community relationships, web site design, web usage tracking and web site configuration.

248

About Mike Reed

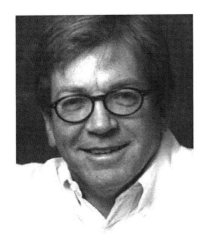

When he first started drawing, Mike Reed drew just to amuse himself.

It wasn't long, though, before he knew he wanted to be an artist.

Today he does illustrations for children's books, for magazines, for catalogs, and for ads.

He also teaches illustration at the College of Visual Art in St. Paul, Minnesota. Mike Reed says, "Making pictures is like acting — you can paint yourself into the action." He often paints on the computer, but he also draws in pen and ink and paints in acrylics. He feels that learning to draw well is the key to being a successful artist.

Mike is regarded as one of the nation's premier illustrators and is the creator of the popular "Flame Warriors" illustrations at **www.flamewarriors.com**. A renowned children's artist, Mike has also provided the illustrations for dozens of children's books.

Mike Reed has always enjoyed reading. As a young child, he liked the Dr. Seuss books. Later, he started reading biographies and war stories. One reason why he feels lucky to be an illustrator is because he can listen to books on tape while he works. Mike is available to provide custom illustrations for all manner of publications at reasonable process. Mike can be reached at **www.mikereedillustration.com**.